Why D
Pediatrician Tell Me That?

Alternative Solutions for
Healthy Growing Families

Dr. Brenda Fairchild

DC, CACCP, BA, BS, RT(R)(M)

DEDICATION

I would like to dedicate this book to my daughter, Madelyn Jaymes, who guided me toward becoming a pregnancy and pediatric chiropractic expert.

I cannot thank my husband, Joseph, and his parents, Ed and Linda, enough for all of their love and support. I have to thank my parents, James and Julie Richey, who watch over us every day, beaming with joy; and my sister, Rebecca, who is always by my side. Kristyn Walters has been there for me from the beginning.

Thank you Kim Johnson, Kate Brown, Anny Sadler, and Caitlyn O'Grady for making this a reality. Finally, I must thank Dr. Claudia Anrig, Dr. Monika Buerger, and ICPA for support and training!

DISCLAIMER

This book is to provide you with information and accurate research to help you make an informed choice when visiting your doctor and to let you know that there are other options out there for your children.

You should never self-diagnose, and you should always work with a physician, whether it be your pediatrician, chiropractor, or a naturopath. I do not receive any compensation from any of the companies mentioned in the book.

These are products I have trusted and have had great results in helping children get well.

CONTENTS

FOREWORD

Being a natural mom and a chiropractor, I felt that this book desperately needed to be written. This book came out of frustration of my personal dealings with my daughter and various pediatricians, what I would hear in these offices, and the frustrations my patients were experiencing with their own pediatricians and doctors.

It seemed as though, in the doctors' eyes, there were no alternatives to mainstream medicine, or they were quick to discredit natural alternatives to helping our children. They seemed to believe that medication was the only way to heal conditions, because that is all some studies show.

It is important to realize that the majority of these studies are released and funded by the pharmaceutical companies who are profiting from every prescription their consumers fill. Never once did a medical professional ask about Madelyn's diet, her water or beverage intake, or whether she was taking any vitamins.

I often received the textbook answer, "We do not recommend vitamins because they are not FDA approved." They only asked about what medicines she was taking.

Is medicine really the sole answer to raising a healthy child? It makes me upset to think about the amount of antibiotics our children are prescribed without even knowing if the illness is even bacterial in nature.

Not only are mainstream doctors over-prescribing antibiotics, but the amount of antibiotics we ingest just from our food is staggering. Viruses are mutating all the time; we now have inadvertently created strains of bacterial superbugs that are resistant to antibiotics. If you have seen the news lately, you have seen that healthy children are dying from the flu. Why?

The title of this book came from my patients, when they were amazed to see how fast, easy, and naturally they could heal their children without medication(s). Simple changes in diet or taking a probiotic made a significant difference in their lives. They would always say to me, "Why didn't my pediatrician tell me that?" My response was always, "You will have to ask them that yourself."

This is my and gift to you and your family. We are letting you in on the other options that are out there to help you. In this book we will talk about everything from diet, nutritional supplements, natural home remedies, immunizations, posture, medical studies, and lack thereof. We know how much these things have helped our children, but I have personally seen them help so many children in my office.

This is about looking at a child as a whole, not

just focusing solely on the symptoms. It's about raising a healthier child overall. I hope that you enjoy this book and find it to be a valuable resource through the various stages of life as your family grows.

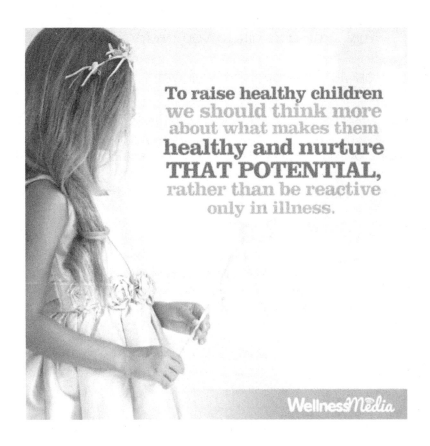

To raise healthy children we should think more about what makes them **healthy and nurture THAT POTENTIAL,** rather than be reactive only in illness.

Wellness&Media

CHAPTER 1

WHY DIDN'T MY PEDIATRICIAN TELL ME ABOUT KEEPING MY CHILD WELL?

I cannot speak for how it is when you go to your pediatrician, but *never* have we ever been asked what we do at home to keep Madelyn healthy. They never asked about her diet, sleeping habits, water intake, if she has had any recent falls, or if she was taking any vitamins. More often than not, I would leave with some sort of prescription, maybe a referral to a specialist, and then I get the vaccine lecture. I would get angry, feeling like we had wasted our time, and we would leave.

According to their "wellness" plan, they suggested I come back (depending on their vaccine schedule) anywhere from 1-6 months later. You mean I am supposed to bring my healthy daughter into an office full of sick children for her "wellness" check? Yes! That sounds like a great idea!

To ease your mind, they tell you they separate sick the children from the well children on different sides of the waiting room. This presupposes that germs don't travel at all, everyone washes their hands, and there are not any germs or fluids on their clothes at all from going back and forth between seeing sick children and well children, of course.

So, after I bring my daughter in for her "wellness" check and inevitably leave with some sort of cold, flu, or fever over the next week, I then have to bring her back to the "sick" side later in the week. If you come in healthy, there is nothing they can prescribe you with. Multi-vitamins are not recommended by the FDA so they will not approve them, but.... Madelyn is due for her MMR, rotavirus and flu shot all full of known neurotoxins.

Ingredients such as thimerosal, aluminum, formaldehyde, as well as fetal cells are ok since they are approved by the FDA. (For a complete list of ingredients, please visit the Center for Disease Control and Prevention at the following website.

www.cdc.gov/vaccines/vac-gen/additives.htm

You and your child are exposed to who-knows-what, and you leave with no less the 3 prescriptions which that they have explained nothing to you. You don't know of any side effects or even if safe to use for children under the age of one. It can be very frustrating to get answers.

Many parents are surprised to learn that they do not have to see a pediatrician. There are many other healthcare providers that can assist in raising a healthy child. You can see a family doctor, a pediatric chiropractor (I see many families as their primary care physician or pediatrician), a naturopath or homeopath, a physician's assistant, or nurse practitioner. All of these medical professionals are specialized in their field and trained in helping to heal your sick child, as well as in assisting to keep your child well.

Medical professionals should be working with you as a team. You should not be looked down upon for the decisions that you make. Whether about homeopathic remedies or your vaccine schedule, you should be supported. It is important to just remember that <u>they work for you</u>.

If you are not seeing eye to eye, then it may be time to move on. It may take you some time to find the right provider for you. But take your time. This is an important decision, and one that should not be taken lightly.

My daughter is hardly ever sick, but when she is, it is a doozy and she is wiped out for few days- and that is okay! Getting sick every now and then is perfectly alright, and is an important part of building a strong immune system. But your kids should not be chronically sick. That is the sign of a weak immune system, and we need to boost it up! So, let's go through some things to Keep Your Children Healthy!

Let's start with some easy things. **Sleep!** Your child needs to get plenty of it.   My recommendations for sleeping:

Infant	18 hours
Toddler	12 hours
School aged	10 hours
Young adult	8-10 hours

Sleep helps us to reset our bodies. When we sleep, our cells regenerate and heal our bodies. Sleep helps in maintaining healthy thyroid and adrenal glands, which are organs essential to controlling your body. You will hear me talk about them many times throughout the book.

I can almost guarantee that you will never hear your pediatrician talk about your child's thyroid. But in my clinical practice, more and more children are developing hypothyroid (underactive thyroid) due to mom being undiagnosed during pregnancy, lack of nutrients, and poor sleeping habits from not only in the womb, but from the onset of birth. Sleeping in infancy sets the tone for life! NEVER wake a sleeping baby to feed. They will eat when they wake up.

Make sure your child is drinking plenty of **water**. Did you know that we are the only mammals to drink milk as adults and we are the only mammal to drink another mammal's milk? If your child is eating a balanced diet, they do not need additional calcium. They should get enough through foods, and, as long as vitamin D levels are in the best functional range (between 60-80ng/mL), your child will be able to properly absorb calcium.

Unfortunately, there are many downsides to the consumption of cow's milk. I have pediatric patients who experience <u>chronic joint pain</u>. The first thing that I suggest is to remove dairy from their diet. Like magic, all aches and pains typically go away. Cow's milk can also lead to constipation and digestive problems. In a recent study conducted in Sweden, they were able to link milk consumption to increased bone fractures and increased mortality (1). I may do a food sensitivity test to see if their body is reactive to milk and other foods.

Water should be your child's primary drink. The rule of thumb for daily water consumption is your child's body weight divided by 2. That means a 50 pound child should be drinking 25 ounces of water per day to stay hydrated. By cutting out cow's milk and keeping your child properly hydrated with water, you will notice fewer aches and pains, hear less complaining of their stomach pain, find your child to be sleeping better, and you will notice how much clearer their skin looks. Pass on the milk, and say yes to water!

Diet is something that many pediatricians do not talk about. Truth be told, this is potentially one of the hardest things to change in your child's life. Raising a picky eater myself, I know the struggles. You don't want to push too hard that they push back and have a lifetime of food phobias. So, it has to be on their terms. At our house, we try to incorporate different new fruits and vegetables every 1-2 weeks and make a big production out of it. And give Maddy lots of praising when she eats something new.

If you can, stick with whole, unprocessed foods, and just do the best you can. If possible, you should try to choose organic or locally grown produce. This will keep down the amount of pesticides. When purchasing meats, look for organic, free range, and grass fed. That means the animals are receiving no grains, no harmful antibiotics, and are hormone free. I always tell my patients to put their organic dollars into meats and dairy. It can be more expensive, but I believe that it is worth it in the long run.

The hormones that are injected into the animals we consume (along with other chemicals and plastics) are causing young girls to reach puberty at an early age(82), and the large amount of antibiotics we are being exposed to through our food and from doctors are causing us to become more resistant to medical antibiotics which can occasionally be necessary.

The CDC (Center for Disease Control and Prevention) states that antibiotics should not be given for colds, flu, cough, or bronchitis (as they are viral), and a big concern from a public health standpoint is bacteria is becoming less responsive to antibiotics. So, antibiotics should only be taken when absolutely needed. (2)

Exercise!!! Get out and play! Our bodies are designed to move. The more movement, the healthier we are. Running, jumping, climbing on jungle gyms, etc., are all great not only for weight control, but exercise also helps to strengthen our mind and bones, helps to drain the lymph system, and helps to get the digestive juices flowing to aid in digestion and better sleep. If you can, try to get outside to exercise. Sunny days are especially great because they help to get natural Vitamin D from the sun and breathe in fresh air.

Fevers. Fevers can be scary, but they are part

of what helps us to stay healthy. We should not be suppressing them, but rather let them do their job. Fevers help to regulate the body and fight off viruses and infections. <u>Fevers are a good thing</u>! According to the American Pediatric Association (APA), the guidelines for healthy fever ranges for a baby 12 weeks or under is considered 100.4 degrees.

Over 12 weeks old to adulthood, a healthy range for a fever is considered under 104 degrees. Somewhere along the line, we have developed a "fever phobia". The best way to help a child with a fever is first and foremost, Let Them Sleep! Do not wake them up, they need rest. Also, keep them hydrated. Offer plenty of water and fluids. As many of you know, most pediatricians want you to alternate ibuprofen and acetaminophen to help reduce fever. Here is the APA stance of alternating therapies:

"...*questions remain regarding the safety of this practice as well as the effectiveness in improving discomfort, which is the primary treatment end point. The possibility is that parents will either not receive or not understand dosing instructions, combined with the wide array of formulations that contain these drugs, increases the potential for inaccurate dosing or overdosing.*"

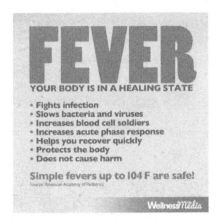

It is best to let the fever ride out, and not to panic: It's just a fever. Your child is not going to feel well, will be lethargic, and not want to eat much. This is normal. It will most likely be over in 24-48 hours. Always keep your child home from school if they have a fever. **Rest is Best!**

Regular **chiropractic adjustments** will help keep your child healthy and, when sick, help to reduce fever by boosting their immune system to help fight colds and flu faster (3). Your nervous system is the master system of your body. It is the first to develop, and every single cell and organ is controlled by the nervous system. You need to take care of your spine. Spinal alignments help to make sure the proper nerve flow is running in the body, free of interference.

Misalignments happen all the time. They can be caused during birth, from falls, traumas, stress, chemicals from what we eat and drink, or from the medicines we take. Your body craves balance. The evidence is right in front of us. We have two arms, two legs, two eyes, two ears, and so on; each placed symmetrically on our body. Looking at the midline of the body, you have only one spine.

When the body is out of balance, this can lead to problems such has behavioral issues, back pain, joint pain, etc., which are due to improper balance of the body. The sooner you start maintaining the balance of the body, the less the chances are of problems in adulthood. **Be proactive about your wellness**.

Regular care of your spine is just as important as going to the dentist. How would your teeth look if you didn't keep up on regular maintenance? Not very good! You have one spine, so take care of it!

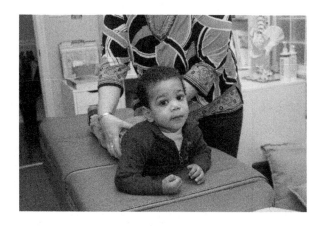

In a study conducted in 1975, Dr. Ronald Pero's team measured 107 individuals who had received long-term chiropractic care. The chiropractic patients were shown to have a 200% greater immune competence than people who had not received chiropractic care. (4)

Even back in 1975, they knew the importance and the power of chiropractic care in keeping you healthy. In another randomized, controlled clinical trial, HIV patients were given an upper cervical adjustment. Those that received the adjustment showed a 48% increase on CD4 cells, while the control saw an 8% decrease. CD4 or T-helper cells are the type of white blood cells which help to fight off infection. Having your body properly aligned will help to increase your white count, and help to boost your immune system. (5) To find a pediatric chiropractor close to you go to www.icpa4kids.org

In addition to water, sleep, regular chiropractic care, and whole foods, you need to support the body with nutrients. Our foods today have become nutrient-poor from the lack of vitamins and minerals in our soil. Because of this, we need to supplement. When purchasing supplements, be sure to purchase pharmaceutical-grade products. You may have heard about the products at stores such as Wal-Mart, Target, and CVS being inferior to their pricier competitors and full of fillers. Some reports show that only 4% of what is listed on the bottle is actually in the product. The New York State Attorney General's office is conducting further investigation of big box store supplements.

Unfortunately, buying the cheapest isn't always the best, and it can provide a false sense of security. Just the other day I had a family who brought in all their supplements, mainly from inexpensive big box stores. Some of them were full of sugar, corn starch, food colorings, and one had wax (and families are concerned why they are not feeling better). When I do lab work on my patients, we often find that they are globally deficient of various vitamins and minerals even though they have a balanced diet and are taking a multivitamin.

The products that I carry in my office are some of the best quality vitamins out there. I use DaVinci Laboratories of Vermont, Apex Energetics, Standard Process, Nordic Naturals, Xymogen, Klaire, Seeking Health, and Thorne. All of these companies have strict regulations and guidelines, and they are not willing to put their reputation on the line. I know the products work because I do lab testing to make sure the patients' bodies are absorbing the nutrients. Be careful when purchasing supplements. Spend a little more money to get a better quality product.

What should your child be taking? Like I said before, I like to do lab work to see the big picture. But if that is not an option, I would have your child on a good multivitamin first and foremost. There are plenty out there to choose from. I usually recommend Nordic Naturals, Klaire, Juice Plus, or Garden of Life. You just have to find one your child likes, and though you may have to go through a few brands until you find one that works for your family.

A healthy child has a healthy gut. **Probiotics**

are a great way to keep your kids healthy. I like kids to be on a broad spectrum probiotic containing a minimum of 7 different strands of bacteria. Probiotics aid in proper digestion, help children to have regular bowel movements, can help with reflux issues, and help to boost the immune system.

Everyone who has taken an antibiotic should be taking probiotics to repopulate the good bacteria, as antibiotics do not discriminate between good and bad bacteria. Taking a probiotic after a round of antibiotics helps to prevent the overgrowth of yeast in the body. I recommend using a powder-form probiotic, some prefer liquid.

I use DaVinci and Klaire brands because they are GMO-, gluten-and dairy-free, and can be given to adults and children alike. There is no taste, so you can add a little to foods and drinks, swab a baby's mouth with it, or if breastfeeding, moms can put it on the nipple so that it mixes with breast milk.

Some parents like live cultures and others like Kefir, which is a tart dairy product that has much more probiotics than yogurt, and some families like Kombucha. You can make your own Kefir or Kombucha, or purchase them in various flavors in stores. It is up to you and your child to decide what works best for you.

You may also want to look into **digestive**

enzymes to aid in digestion. They help to break down sugars, carbohydrates, and milk. Because of our often highly processed food diets, the enzymes in our body have a harder time breaking down the foods we eat. Because of this, our bodies are not absorbing nutrients properly. Over time, foods that are not broken down can begin to seep into our blood, causing what is referred to as "leaky gut." Long term, this condition can lead to autoimmune disorders such as Crohn's disease, Lupus, or Hashimoto's.

There are many different digestive enzymes, but here we will touch on the major ones. Each enzyme plays a role in breaking down the foods we eat.

- Lipase = fat

- Protease = proteins

- Amylases = carbohydrates

- Lactase = Milk

Taking digestive enzymes in addition to probiotics will help boost the immune system, and will help your child to use the bathroom on a regular basis.

Depending on where you live, you may have to supplement with **Vitamin D**. If you live in a sunnier part of the country, you may not have to, but otherwise it is likely that you will need to. I prefer liquid Vitamin D. Here in the office, we use Xymogen brand. I have been very pleased with results, and patient feedback has been very positive.

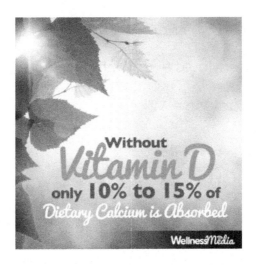

I follow the guidelines of the Vitamin D Council (6) which states that children should be getting 1,000-2,000 IU's per day depending on age and weight. If mom is breastfeeding, she can take 5,000-10,000 IU's per day, on average. Vitamin D will pass through breast milk according to the Vitamin D Council, so there is no need to supplement the baby if the mother is supplementing.

The best way to get natural vitamin D is from the sun. On a bright sunny day, get outside for 10-20 minutes without sunscreen between the hours of 12:00 noon to 2:00 PM. Expose as much skin as possible to maximize absorption not only with vitamin D but with calcium as well. This is great for the whole family including babies.

Another supplement to consider is **magnesium.** It tends to be a silent deficiency because it is harder to detect, and blood levels may not always show a deficiency. Signs of low magnesium can be constipation, sleeplessness, restless leg, chronic pain or fibromyalgia, brain fog, and difficulty concentrating.

Daily recommendations are 500-1,000mg per day. I have children start on the lower end, 100-200mg, and see how they respond. Too much magnesium can cause diarrhea, so you have to be careful. It is important to start slowly with a smaller dosage. I like to combine magnesium with **CoQ10**. CoQ10 is an antioxidant and it is needed to provide the energy for cells to function properly. It is great for the heart, helps fight off fatigue, and many athletes use it to recover from workouts and support muscles and bones.

Vitamin C is always great to help boost the immune system, especially in the winter months.

It is a great way to keep cold and flu away, or to help get over it faster. Vitamin C is found in mainly fruits and vegetables, but if you have a picky eater, you may need to supplement. According to the National Institutes of Health (NIH), the recommendations for children are: (7)

- Infants 0-6 months old, 40 mg per day
- Infants 7-12 months old, 50 mg per day
- 1–3 years 15 mg
- 4–8 years 25 mg
- 9–13 years 45 mg
- 14–18 years 65-75 mg
- 19+ years 75-90 mg

I tend to recommend higher doses from 325-

1,000 mg per day, and definitely higher doses when sick. Just like magnesium, taking too much can produce diarrhea, so be on the lookout.

Make sure you don't forget the Omega's or fish oil. You can either do a blend or you can stick with an Omega 3. It is up to you. There are many benefits to fatty acids, they help a child's developing brain, heart health, aids in bowel regulation, helps with autoimmunity, and can help with skin, hair, and nails. Everyone should be taking a high-quality Omega. This is not a supplement you want to go inexpensive on. Buy a good one. One of my favorite companies is Nordic Naturals. They are the gold standard when it comes to Omegas.

Many people do not know they should also be taking a **mineral complex**. Most of our multivitamins, even the best ones, have around 10 different minerals at most. We should be getting upwards of 70-80 minerals daily. Our lack of minerals is leading us down the path of thyroid issues, fertility problems in men and women, and higher autoimmunity conditions.

A mineral complex should be part of your child's supplement regiment. I recommend a liquid variety, specifically Cheri-Mins from Youngevity. Many of my patients are concerned when they see the minerals lead, nickel, and silver. These are all trace minerals, and our bodies actually need them. They are also found in our soil, so if you are eating plant-based foods, you are ingesting these minerals. So when you see these ingredients, don't panic.

Now is the time to address the elephant in the room: Vaccines. While there is no denying that they work in most cases, they are not one-size-fits-all. And though they are meant to protect you against viruses, they often mutate and have different strains, so you may not be fully protected as we have seen recently with the flu vaccine. We are here to address the health and wellbeing of your child, and vaccines and immunizations are an important topic of that discussion.

Choosing whether or not to vaccinate your

child is not an easy decision to make, and should not be taken lightly. I always advise my patients to educate themselves as much as possible before making a decision. Doctors often do not voluntarily or truthfully inform you of what is in the actual vaccines, nor do they mention the multitude of possible side effects.

Ask to see the insert and have your pediatrician discuss the ingredients, side effects, the health of you and your child along with food possible food allergies because it all goes hand in hand. Many parents do not know some vaccines are made with eggs. So if you have a child allergic to eggs, vaccines may not agree with them and cause more harm than good.

Should your child have a reaction to the vaccine, your pediatrician and the manufacturing company are both protected by the government, whereas your child is the one suffering the sometimes life-changing or fatal consequences of the vaccine. It is up to you to make the best-informed choice for your child and your family. You should be educated on the ingredients and on the pros and cons of vaccinating. Know what they are good for, and also be aware of the side effects.

EDUCATION IS POWER! As a parent, you do have options. You can do full schedule as the CDC recommends, you can delay and/or do a partial schedule, or you have the option not to vaccinate at all. The decision is yours. It is important to remember <u>you can never un-vaccinate</u>.

Regardless of your decision, finding a doctor who is willing to support you, your family, and your choices, is of the utmost importance. Take your time and find the right doctor for your needs.

If you would like to learn more, here are some of my favorite books and websites to explore:

- <u>www.nvic.org</u>
- <u>www.cdc.gov/vaccines</u>
- The Vaccine Book by Dr. Sears
- Vaccine Epidemic by Habakus & Holland
- What Your Doctor May Not Tell You

About Children's Vaccinations by Stephanie Cave

- Vaccines, Autism, and Chronic Inflammation: The New Epidemic by Barbara Loe Fisher

- Bought http://www.boughtmovie.com/

- Trace Amounts http://traceamounts.com/

- Doctored http://www.doctoredthemovie.com/

I have many parents who choose to vaccinate but are not sure they want to follow the schedule. Many parents are unsure of the timeline when their child may need a booster shot. You can have a **titer** done to see if a booster is needed. Most pediatricians will not offer you this option outright, but it can be done through lab work.

You can also order it on your own at www.directlabs.com/tenpenny/OrderTests/tabid/13150/language/en-US/Default.aspx.

The titer will show you if the patient has antibodies to a particular vaccine like MMR, Hib, or DtaP. If the titer comes back high, the patient does not need a booster, but if it is low and you are following the CDC's schedule, then the patient will need to get the booster shot. Don't be afraid to speak up and ask for the titer.

Remember, your doctor works for you. On a follow-up note, there are not any studies verifying the efficacy of the schedule. The CDC recommends 49 doses of 14 vaccines by the age of 6 and 69 doses by the age of 18. (8)

TABLE 1. Recommended schedule for active immunization of normal infants and children (See individual ACIP recommendations for details.)

Recommended age*	Vaccine(s)[†]	Comments
2 mo.	DTP-1,[§] OPV-1[¶]	Can be given earlier in areas of high endemicity
4 mo.	DTP-2, OPV-2	6-wks-2-mo. interval desired between OPV doses to avoid interference
6 mo.	DTP-3	An additional dose of OPV at this time is optional for use in areas with a high risk of polio exposure
15 mo.**	MMR[††]	
18 mo.**	DTP-4, OPV-3	Completion of primary series
4-6 yr.[§§]	DTP-5, OPV-4	Preferably at or before school entry
14-16. yr	Td[¶¶]	Repeat every 10 years throughout life

*These recommended ages should not be construed as absolute, i.e. 2 mos. can be 6-10 weeks, etc.
[†]For all products used, consult manufacturer's package enclosure for instructions for storage, handling, and administration. Immunobiologics prepared by different manufacturers may vary, and those of the same manufacturer may change from time to time. The package insert should be followed for a specific product.
[§]DTP—Diphtheria and tetanus toxoids and pertussis vaccine.
[¶]OPV—Oral, attenuated poliovirus vaccine contains poliovirus types 1, 2, and 3.
**Simultaneous administration of MMR, DTP, and OPV is appropriate for patients whose compliance with medical care recommendations cannot be assured.
[††]MMR—Live measles, mumps, and rubella viruses in a combined vaccine (see text for discussion of single vaccines versus combination).
[§§]Up to the seventh birthday.
[¶¶]Td—Adult tetanus toxoid and diphtheria toxoid in combination, which contains the same dose of tetanus toxoid as DTP or DT and a reduced dose of diphtheria toxoid.

1983 childhood immunization schedule

(80)

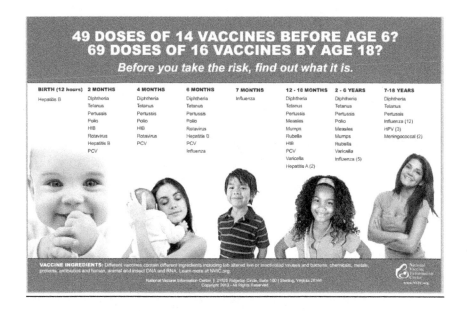

Source: The National Vaccine Information Center (NVIC) is a charitable non-profit organization founded in 1982 to prevent vaccine injuries and deaths through public education and the inclusion of informed consent protections in public health vaccine policies and laws. This graphic representation of the CDC's recommended childhood vaccine schedule appears with NVIC's permission and can be accessed at http://www.nvic.org/CMSTemplates/NVIC/pdf/49-Doses-PosterB.pdf. Its use does not imply NVIC's endorsement of statements or opinions in this publication.

Should your child have a reaction, please make sure it is reported. You can go to Vaccine Adverse Event Reporting System (VAERS) online: http://www.vaers.hhs.gov. Here you can list what kind of a reaction your child experienced.

There is so much more that we could go into, but the links and books should get you started if you would like to further research vaccines. Before we move on to the next topic, I do want to leave you with a bit of information on T-helper cells to give you a better understanding of why unvaccinated children tend to be more healthy, versus vaccinated children who tend to have higher occurrences of allergies, eczema, or asthma.

T-helper cells are involved in our adaptive immunity. They help us to fight off bacteria and other viruses that we come in contact with. We should have an even balance of Th1/Th2 cells. T helper 1 (Th1) help to fight off bacteria, viruses, and cancers from inside the cells, otherwise known as our cellular immunity. When a child is exposed to illnesses such as chicken pox or measles, their bodies elicit a Th1 response and give a child a lifetime of immunity.

T helper 2 (Th2) are activated to fight off extracellular parasites, (including vaccines) and is described as humoral immunity. If there is too much Th1 you can have a delay in skin reactions. If a person has a high Th2 ratio, this can cause symptoms like a constant runny nose, eczema, allergies, and asthma, as well as autoimmune diseases (9) (10). Does this sound familiar?

Vaccinated children have a high ratio of Th2

over Th1, which is why some are prone to chronic illness. Many of my patients' parents follow pediatrician Robert W. Sears, MD, who suggests an alternate schedule, explained in his book *The Vaccine Book: Making the Right Decision for Your Child*. I also have others who choose to veer from the suggested schedule by having one vaccine given at a time, with 1-2 months between each injection. This way, should their child have a reaction, they are able to easily identify which vaccine caused the reaction.

Whichever route you choose to take, be sure to find a pediatrician who is willing to work with your and your family's choices. Should you decide to vaccinate, it is important to get their systems balanced again and to do what we previously discussed: probiotics, omega 3's, and minerals containing selenium and zinc (mineral complex is best). (9) (10)

The best thing you can do when considering vaccinations is to educate yourself. Seek out a doctor who is supportive of your decisions, and explore peer groups, as well. There are many social groups full of like-minded people, as well as other parents looking to further educate themselves.

You also may want to consider joining the Holistic Moms Network www.holisticmoms.org/, and finding a chapter close to where you live. There are lots of families that will support and share in your decisions for raising your family. You have rights, and you have the option to opt out of vaccines entirely if you so choose. As always, the decision is up to you and your family.

.

No one said raising a healthy is easy, and it is normal to feel overwhelmed at times. I struggle with it myself. My pediatrician and I do not always see eye to eye on all of my decisions, but I know my daughter best, just as you know your children better than anyone. Trust your gut. No matter your choice, you are making the best decision for your child, and the point of this book is to aid you in making choices along the way.

Be proud of yourself! You are doing an amazing job at raising your children, and by reading this book, you are educating yourself about alternative, natural choices that you pediatrician may not tell you about. There are endless options out there, and I am sharing a large portion of them with you in this text.

Quick Reference for Wellness

1. Sleep

2. Water

3. Diet

4. Chiropractic care

5. Multivitamins

6. Probiotic/digestive enzymes

7. Magnesium

8. Vitamin C

9. Multi-minerals

10. Vitamin D

11. Omega 3's

12. Vaccine-Informed Decision

13. Titers

14. Like-minded Peer Groups

CHAPTER 2

WHY DIDN'T MY PEDIATRICIAN TELL ME ABOUT OTHER OPTIONS FOR COLIC?

For the exhausted, sleep-deprived parent, a colic diagnosis can feel like the end of the world. In today's society, colic is annotated as an endless, helpless, miserable experience, leaving parents and their babies feeling completely defeated. Though colic is a difficult thing for everyone involved, there is hope. Despite what many doctors say, there are solutions to help you and your baby through this difficult time.

The definition of colic came from pediatrician Dr. Morris Wessel over 40 years ago. It is now most easily diagnosed based on the "Rule of 3's": A child who cries more than 3 hours a day for more than 3 days a week, over 3 consecutive weeks is deemed colicky.

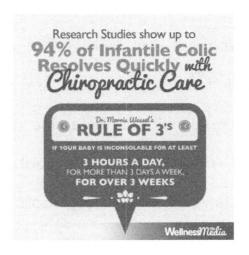

This also applies only after baby has been changed, burped, swaddled, made comfortable, bounced, patted gently on their bottom, and if you have already removed dairy or soy from your diet, but the baby continues to cry. You may have changed from one formula to another, and possibly even back to the original formula, and found nothing but frustration. You may notice the baby arching their back, jutting their legs straight and outward, not wanting to be touched or held, having a hard belly, exhibiting signs of reflux, and fashioning a constant pained, grimaced facial expression.

Some parents say their baby seems perfectly fine during the day, but then seems to get fussy at night, usually at the same time each day. It goes without saying that colic is a very unpleasant experience for everyone involved.

The fastest way to resolve colic is to get your

child to a **pediatric chiropractor** as soon as possible. You can find one in your area by going to icpa4kids.org/. Colic is caused by outside conditions while the baby is still in the womb. Excessive sitting, lack of exercise, and a processed diet void of vitamins and minerals can be to blame. I often see colic, in breech, and transverse babies from mothers who spent a lot of time at the computer while pregnant. These conditions can cause intrauterine constraint and can limit the amount of room the baby has to develop. This is why chiropractic adjustments during pregnancy are extremely important to the development of your baby.

Arching of the back is a sign of tight muscles or

can be a sign of gastrointestinal issues such as reflux, gas, or possible food sensitivities. Feel your baby's head; you may notice ridges one side of the head but not the other. Many children with colic sometimes have an undiagnosed case of torticollis, where they are always looking to one side, and fuss when your try to turn their head the other way. Some babies have an aversion to tummy-time or frequent crying in their car seat are often signs of spinal and skull misalignments, as well as muscle imbalances.

An adjustment on a baby is much different than that of an adult, but has the same premise. I use only my finger tip and the amount of pressure used is the same if you were to press your finger through a ripe tomato: so very little pressure. Babies do not have the same stresses we have as adults, so a light adjustment is all that is needed. Because of this, babies usually respond to care much faster than adult patients.

A randomized, controlled trial at the Center for Biomechanics at Odense University in Denmark found that chiropractic adjustments on infants reduced crying by up to 2.7 hours, as compared to the group that was given dimethicone; the active anti-foaming agent ingredient in many colic drops to help reduce gas. It can also be found in hair products to make your hair shiny as it is considered a silicon oil.   You will see it called Simethicone in colic drops or in some anti-acids to help with bloating. The dimethicone group only saw a decrease in colic by 1 hour and saw no improvement thereafter (11).

Another study, a pragmatic single-blind, randomized controlled trial of 104 babies with colic, saw a decrease in crying up to 2 hours with chiropractic care. The conclusion: "In this study, chiropractic manual therapy improved crying behavior in infants with colic. The findings showed that knowledge of treatment by the parent did not appear to contribute to the observed treatment effects in this study. Thus, it is unlikely that observed treatment effect is due to bias on the part of the reporting parent. (12)

A 2011 review of available literature resulted in the following findings: "Our systematic review of the literature revealed 26 articles meeting our inclusion criteria. These consisted of three clinical trials, two survey studies, six case reports, two case series, four cohort studies, five commentaries, and four reviews of the literature. Our findings reveal that chiropractic care is a viable alternative to the care of infantile colic and congruent with evidence-based practice, particularly when one considers that <u>medical care options are no better than placebo or have associated adverse events (13)</u>."

A prospective, uncontrolled study of 316 infants suffering from infantile colic and selected according to well-defined criteria shows a **satisfactory result of spinal manipulative therapy in 94% of the cases.** The median age of the infants was 5.7 weeks at the beginning of the treatment. The results were evaluated by analysis of a diary continuously kept by the mother and an assessment file comprised by interview. The study was carried out as a multicenter study lasting 3 months and involving 73 chiropractors in 50 clinics. The results occurred within 2 weeks and after an average of three treatments. (74)

Typically I begin to see a difference within 1-2 weeks of starting care. Families are amazed by how fast the adjustments start to help their little ones. Parents generally notice an immediate change in their child's sleep and continue to see how much of a difference chiropractic care makes in reducing crying time. Many pediatricians have now begun to recommend antacids, histamine, or H2 blockers for their "silent reflux" as they like to call it. Most of the families who have come in said they did not see any improvement when these were introduced.

I am always concerned when I hear they told their pediatrician the H2 blockers did not work because I know they will be prescribed something stronger like a proton pump inhibitor or PPI. These help to block the secretion of acid in the stomach. This then leads to food not being properly digested because of the lack of acid, and then this can lead to constipation and now your child will have to be put on another medication to help them move their bowels. In addition, all of these medications can cause B12 or cobalamin to not be absorbed. Long term this can lead to chronic fatigue, depression, not sleeping, and so on. So, as you can see it follows a vicious cycle. I talk more about these topics in the reflux and constipation chapters.

Often with colic, there are accompanying digestive problems, including gas, reflux, or constipation, so we need to work on the gut, as well. Some parents try using a product called Gripe water, but the results often vary. If it works for you, fantastic! My go-to is always

aloe juice. This will help to calm down an irritated or gassy belly in no time. I recommend this for babies who have reflux and are experiencing constipation, too. Aloe juice helps gets things moving. Just as aloe soothes a sunburn, it will soothe the lining of the bowel, as well. Calming down the stomach acid allows more nutrients to be absorbed, in turn reducing baby's fussiness and helping you both get some sleep.

For an infant, I recommend giving 1-2mL of aloe juice once in the morning, and once at night. For best results, try serving it on an empty stomach, but that may not always be feasible, so just do the best you can. Try first using a syringe, but if you need to, adding the juice to a bottle is perfectly fine. You may want to look for an aloe juice that has some flavoring to reduce the chance of your baby spitting it out. Unflavored aloe juice has a bitter flavor, and most adults do not like the taste either. There may be some sugar added, but I personally feel that the benefits outweigh the sugar in this instance.

Since many times reflux and colic many times go hand-in-hand, I have parents focus on the **cardiac sphincter**, which is located below the breastbone. This is a valve that connects the esophagus to the stomach. In many babies, the valve is not mature enough to function properly and can be a major cause of acid reflux by allowing too much gas to enter the stomach.

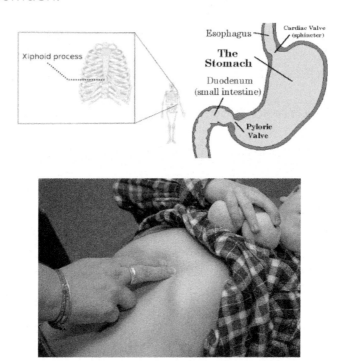

This treatment is simple but effective. Using your finger tip, put one finger just below the xiphoid process, the tip or end of the breastbone, and you will feel a soft spot; that is where you will find the cardiac sphincter. Your baby may fuss or cry at first because it is tender and inflamed.

Rest assured, this reaction will go away within a few days.

Gently hold pressure by pressing down about ¼" and pushing downward towards your child's feet in a scooping motion. Hold sustained pressure for about 10 seconds after every feeding, and when you notice baby spitting up a lot. Doing this will help to stimulate the valve, causing it to close off and block the acid from coming back up.

Vitamin D is also important for a colicky baby. You can either give it to your baby alone as a supplement, or if you are breastfeeding, mom can take it and pass it through her breast milk. (14)(88) According to the Vitamin D Council, infants should be getting up to 1,000 IU's per day, and a lactating mother can take up to 6-10,000 IU's per day. These figures are a far cry from what The Food and Nutrition Board suggests only recommending 600 IU's per adult. With standards like those, it is no wonder we are so deficient in society.

If you live in a warm climate area, like Florida, California, or Las Vegas, etc. you are probably getting plenty of Vitamin D from the sun. Otherwise, you likely need to supplement. In addition to supplementing, the Vitamin D you get from being outside in the sun does wonders for your body. Expose your little one to the sunlight, too, just long enough to get some of that precious "sunshine vitamin." And the fresh air never hurt anyone either.

In addition to what we've mentioned so far, I usually recommend **probiotics** to help babies overcome colic. Look for a probiotic that has 7-10 strains of different bacteria.

Here is a list of a few different strains:

- Lactobacillus acidophilus
- Lactobacillus rhamnosus
- Bifidobacterium lactis
- Lactobacillus casei
- Bifidobacterium Breve
- Bifidobacterium Longum
- Bifidobacterium Bifidum
- Streptococcus thermophiles

If breastfeeding, mom can take them to pass the benefits on to the baby. The baby can also take them as well, just in very small amounts. I recommend using the same probiotic for adults and children, the baby just gets the amount of a finger, see below.

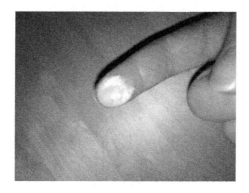

Until their colic is gone, it should be given to baby daily. Once it is over, they should continue to take it at least 2-3 times per week. When first introducing it, you may notice that your baby is actually slightly fussier or gassier. This tells me they needed some good bacteria in their belly. Once they have a good bowel movement, the gas and much of the fussiness will calm down. If the gas continues, you can press on the **ileocecal valve** to help move the gas and stimulate the bowel.

The ileocecal valve is where the small and large intestine meet. If your baby's belly is hard and they are gassy or constipated, the valve is likely stuck closed. Stimulating the valve will help to open it up. The valve is located next to the right hip, and it is only on the right side.

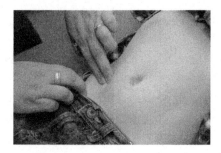

Once you find the hip, move slightly inward toward the belly so that your finger is off of the bone. You will feel tissue there. Apply slight pressure with one finger, pressing down about ¼", and motion upward toward the head in a scooping motion. Hold sustained pressure for a few seconds.

You may feel or hear gurgling, and baby may pass gas or possibly have a bowel movement when you do this. This is good! It is relieving the pressure and cleansing the gut. If your baby's belly is really hard, it may be hard to feel at first.

Go through the motions. More than likely, you have found the right spot. It may be sore and painful for them, so don't be alarmed if they cry a bit. Pain here is a sign the valve is inflamed, but it will get better as the gut heals.

Over the next few days, as the belly becomes softer, they should not be in any pain when you do the maneuver. You do not have to do this all the time. I usually only recommend this technique if baby's belly is hard, or if they are constipated or gassy, but it also works for diarrhea. Adults can use this trigger point method on themselves, as well.

If you are bottle feeding your baby, which type of bottle are you using? Do you hear a lot of air moving in and out of the bottle, or see a lot of bubbles? Does your child cry a lot after feedings? You may need to change your bottle. I always recommend Dr. Brown's bottles to my parents. While the bottles do have a lot of parts to them, it is by far the most superior bottle out there when it comes to avoiding air trapped in your child's belly.

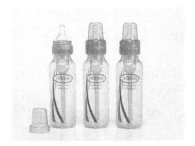

The internal vent helps to create a vacuum and stops air from going back into the bottle, in turn avoiding oxidizing the milk and preserving nutrients. I have personally used these bottles and recommend them often. Most parents notice a huge difference and a decrease of gas and colic.

Try **belly massage**. Babies love contact! When doing belly massage, you will want to go in a clockwise direction using your fingers. You can do in one sweeping motion, or you can go in small circles by pushing air out still moving in the clockwise direction. This will help to relax the muscles, help calm the baby, and relax the bowels.

It will also help to move any gas out that may be trapped. You can do over clothes or on bare skin. If you would like, you can use some essential oils such as lavender or many

companies have their own blend for digestion.
It is up to your discretion.

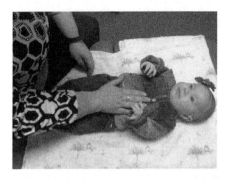

Put your baby on your chest **skin to skin**, this
can help to relax a colicky child, and make
them feel safe and protected, just like they
were in-utero. Our bodies are amazing! You
baby's temperature will regulate to yours. I like
to give this task to dads. Many dads feel left
out if mom is breastfeeding, this gives them a
chance to bond with baby and mom can take
a little nap, a bath, or even better going to the
store all alone!

You can also try wearing your baby. I go more in-depth in the Posture chapter, but babies love to be held and be close to mom and dad. Babies that are worn are happier children and love the security. You will not spoil your baby. There is such a thing as the 4th trimester, this will be discussed more in-depth in my next book, and babies are used to being in tight close spaces. That is why some babies like swaddling. It is what they are used to and know.

When you are wearing your baby, they can hear your heartbeat, a sound they are familiar with since they have been listening to it for months, this will relax them. Wearing is also a healthy way to develop their spine, muscles, organs, as well as a sense of security. Also, the upright position can help if your baby has a tight tummy from gas, holding vertical will take the pressure off the tummy to calm them down.

Just as with anything, there is never just one way to help babies and colic. You have to find what works best for you. Getting your baby adjusted and working on the microbiome will be the most beneficial to helping your little one overcome colic so you and your family can have a more enjoyable experience in raising your infant.

Quick Reference for Colic

1. Pediatric Chiropractic Adjustments

2. Aloe Juice

3. Probiotics

4. Vitamin D

5. Trigger Points

6. Dr. Brown's Bottles

7. Belly Massage

8. Skin to Skin

9. Baby Wearing

CHAPTER 3

WHY DIDN'T MY PEDIATRICIAN TELL ME ABOUT OTHER WAYS TO HELP WITH CONSTIPATION?

(CO-WRITTEN WITH KATIE BROWN BA,SBD,CLD,CCE)

Constipation has become an epidemic in America, not only in children but in adults as well. So, what is causing these belly problems and dysbiosis (microbial imbalance)? Why are we not pooping as a nation? There are so many factors that come into play, and what works for one family may not work for another. Read on to learn how to help your child poop from infancy through potty training.

Did you know we should be having bowel

movements 2-3 times per day, not 2-3 times per week or month like I hear all the time from many parents about their kids? Babies should be moving their bowels 5-8 times per day. Most parents don't know that a baby pooping only once per day is not normal or healthy. You may have heard the gut referred to as your "second brain", and that would be correct. Gut health is so important that about 85% of your immunity comes from your gut. So it goes without saying that we need to take care of our bodies and fuel the digestive tract with the right nutrients to keep things flowing.

Most have not heard of the Enteric Nervous System. It is made up of over 100 million neurons that control your digestive tract.

Believe it or not, the ENS actually contains more neurons than you spinal cord. It responds to emotions and is connected to your brain, which is where the term "second brain" comes from. When you are in love, you may feel "butterflies" in your stomach; when you are about to give a speech, you may get a nervous stomach and may need to "run" to the bathroom; when you get stressed, you may not want to eat, and in turn, your bowels seize up and you may not go for days.

As Americans, we tend to lead busy, stressful lives. We often find ourselves lacking the time to prepare healthy meals, so we go for fast food or pre-packaged foods, which are full of harmful preservatives. Factor in our lack of exercise and it is easy to see the cause of the increase in constipation in our nation.

I have many patients, some as young as two weeks old, who came into my office having been prescribed laxatives or stool softeners for their constipation. The most popular laxative prescribed by pediatricians is actually a wax that helps to keep fluid in your stool so that it can pass more easily. It is intended for short-term use, and should not be used in adults for longer than 7 days. It is not FDA approved in children under 16 years old. The FDA is in the process of doing further studies (87). I have young patients who are actually addicted to it because they have been on it for years. It will take some time to retrain the bowels, and there will be some periods of constipation, but diet is the key. Give it some time, and you can fix your child's bowel issues.

For **infants** with constipation, we do tend to see more than in those who are formula-fed, though that is not always the case. If a baby who is exclusively being breastfeed is having constipation issues, then I have to look at mom and see how her bowels are. Is she pooping 2-3 times a day? Is she having or did have reflux or constipation during pregnancy? Did mom take antibiotics during pregnancy? Did mom do a high quality prenatal (you would be surprised by the number of mom's who do not even take a prenatal vitamin)?

All of these things let me know what is happening with mom and can lead to tummy issues with their baby. A healthy gut of a baby starts in the womb. We will talk about wellness prenatal care in my next book.

An infant should be pooping a minimum of 5-8 times per day. A breastfed baby's stool should look seedy, is usually a mustard yellow color, and is small and soft. A formula-fed infant's poop may be brown, is usually soft, but not always, and usually will have an odor. As you start to introduce solid foods, the texture and smell will change.

Unsure if your baby is constipated?

1. Is their belly hard?

2. Are they grunting a lot?

3. Are they fussy after feedings?

4. Do they arch their back often?

5. Does laying on their tummy seem painful?

6. Are they gassy?

7. Are they having a single bowel movement each day, or none at all)?

8. Do they seem to not like being in their car seat?

9. Do they have reflux? (discussed in later chapter)

If your child is exhibiting any of these symptoms, I suggest that the first thing I do is work on the **ileocecal valve**. The valve is where the small and the large intestines meet. The valve can get stuck open and then you have diarrhea and can be closed which causes can cause constipation.

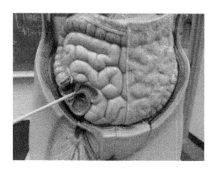

You will want to stimulate the valve to get things moving. Initially, it may be tender and they may cry or fuss the first few times you press on it. It is located ONLY on the right side of the body and it is close to the hip or ilium. For a baby, you will find the hip and move your finger about a ½ inch inward and you will put pressure down and then upward in a scooping motion and hold sustained pressure. Hold pressure for about 30 seconds or so. If there is a lot of gurgling in the belly, then hold until you don't feel or hear anymore. If it is painful, do for a few seconds off and on. The tenderness will start to go away after a few times of releasing the trigger point.

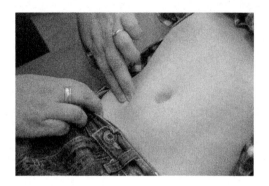

Next we need to start introducing what I call my "GI cocktail" **probiotics** and **aloe juice**. Mom can either directly take the probiotics if she is breastfeeding, or she can give them separately to the baby. Make sure there are at least 7-10 strains of different bacteria. You can either get a powder or a liquid, it's all on what you prefer. Powder tends to be easier if giving to a baby because you can take a pinch and put it in the bottle or on the nipple or swab their mouth with it. More is not always better. Probiotics given once a day should be sufficient.

Next we will give the infant the **aloe juice**. This will help with inflammation of the bowel and help the probiotics to work more effectively. Aloe does wonders for the digestive tract. You will notice your child's belly will be much softer and will start going on a regular basis. Here are the dosages I typically recommend. You will do this **2 times a day** till the constipation is resolved. If you are able, you want to try to have them take it on an empty stomach if possible: first thing in the morning and last thing before bedtime.

Infants 0-5 months	1-2 ML
6 months to 1 year	3-5 ML
Toddlers up to age 5	1-2 ounces
6 – 10 years	2 ounces
11-13 years	3 ounces
14- adult	4 ounces

Most parents see results within 2-3 weeks. I have been recommending aloe juice for years with great results and it is to be in the short term use. There are few studies on aloe and digestion, and further studies need to be conducted (20).

Other supplements to get things moving are

magnesium (citrate or malate). I don't usually start with giving babies magnesium right off the bat. If mom is breastfeeding, I may have her take some. Dosing is hard for babies and not always consistent. I tend to have parents give their little ones Epsom salt baths. The magnesium in the salts will absorb through the skin and help to relax the bowel. I usually start with ¼ cup for babies and up to 1-2 cups for adults in a bathtub. Some parents also like to add lavender as well. That is completely up to you. For toddlers to teenagers, I will have them supplement some magnesium.

Since lab tests may not always give consistent results, it is easier to assume that if they are not going on a regular basis, then they likely have a deficiency. I always start with a small dose and titrate up. As with many things, too much can cause diarrhea. Take it slow. Once again, more is not always better.

Digestive enzymes (DE) are always good to try as well. Most of my parents say the see great results and I have seen great results with my own daughter who struggled with constipation. To me, I feel like these changed our life not only by providing bowel relief, but also by improving mental clarity. DE's help to break down foods so they are more easily absorbed into the bowel so that your body can utilize the vitamins and minerals in the foods.

Because we eat multiple food groups at a time

along with foods being processed, our own enzymes need some help, and that is where DE's come into play. If mom is breastfeeding, I would have her take the supplement. I don't always supplement babies right away, but if I do, I only suggest small doses in their formula. For toddlers to teenagers, they can take them with every meal. I like Klaire's Vital-Zymes others like Thorne or Seeking Health you can't go wrong with any of these brands.

Also, please do not forget to supplement with **vitamin D**. Mom can take up to 5,000 IU and infant can take up to 1,000 IU per day. Vitamin D is much needed for the developing body and helps with aiding in thyroid health which can help with having regular bowel movements. I have noticed a pattern where moms who were deficient in Vitamin D (below 50 mcg in lab work) tend to have babies with more digestive issues. Make sure your doctors are running labs and supplement if need be.

Make sure your baby is getting plenty of tummy time. The more the belly softens, the more they will enjoy being on their front. Tummy time helps to stimulate the brain and can aid in digestion. When on their tummy, you can also stimulate the ileocecal valve. As they are laying there, take 2 fingers and press upwards stimulating the valve. While your baby is doing tummy time, make sure they are moving each of their legs independently.

If they are moving their legs together or not at all, this could signify the misalignment of the pelvis and sacrum, which can hinder development and cause motor delays. If you notice this, please get your child to a **pediatric chiropractor** as soon as possible. The misalignments can also be causing constipation and digestion problems for the baby.

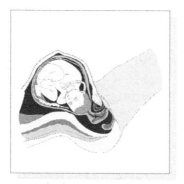

Cephalic presentation

In the womb, the baby is folded and compacted, and the pressure of the tight space can cause misalignments in the head, neck, and lower back. Gentle chiropractic adjustments can realign the body to help increase nerve and blood flow to the bowel, to aid in regular movement.

A case study presented here demonstrated that chiropractic care not only increased the frequency of bowel movements in constipated children, but that the stools were "described as soft without the accompanying straining, pain and rectal bleeding." (83)

Chiropractic America describes in easy-to-understand terms how chiropractic care helps relieve both the symptoms and some of the underlying causes of constipation:

"Chiropractic adjustments (particularly in the lower spine) may help relieve constipation in certain individuals. Muscles in the intestine push stool to the anus, where stool leaves the body. Special nerve cells in the intestine, called ganglion cells, make the muscles push. These nerves connect directly to the celiac ganglion, which also innervate the stomach, liver, gallbladder, spleen, kidney, small intestine, and the ascending and transverse colon. The celiac ganglion, in turn, connects to the spinal cord (and the brain) through nerve roots that exit the spine in the lower thoracic and upper lumbar region. Pressure on these nerve roots caused by misalignment of the vertebrae in this area may interfere with the normal function of the bowel as well as other organs of the digestive system."

You can also stimulate the bowel by doing **bicycle movements**. Have you baby lay on their back and move their legs in a circular movement, like they are pedaling a bike.

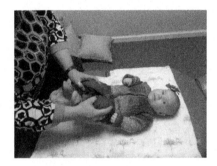

This will help with removing excess gas and getting things moving. After the bicycle, you can rub the baby's tummy in a clockwise motion while using your thumb to put slight pressure on the ileocecal valve and your fingers are moving in a clockwise direction. This will also aid in gas and movement.

If breastfeeding an infant, you may want to remove or greatly limit dairy, as this is known to increase constipation. Eat a diet rich in fruits and vegetables, and drink plenty of water. Also, a diet rich in healthy fish will help provide necessary **Omega 3's**, which help to soften the stool.

If you are not a fish eater, you can certainly supplement with fish oils. I usually recommend Nordic Naturals, but there are plenty of companies out there with high standards who put out a quality product. Don't just pick one off the shelf, ask around and do some research.

Don't forget about **coconut oil**. It has an unbelievable number of benefits. In this case, I like it for its gut-cleansing properties. It helps yeast and candida die off. Adding coconut oil to your diet also helps to keep the bowel moving by keeping it properly hydrated. You can eat it by itself, add it while cooking, or add to smoothies. I usually recommend 2 tablespoons per day. This can also help maintain good cholesterol.

As your child grows, it is important to keep them well hydrated with **pure water**. Children who drink lots of juice and milk will likely have more problems going to the bathroom. These drinks cause hard stools, causing poops to be painful. This can be especially detrimental during potty training, as this can cause children to try to avoid pooping because of the pain. I have seen this firsthand with my own daughter. I recall many times that she would cry in pain, but once we cut out the milk and substituted water, she started going on a more regular basis.

The rule of thumb regarding daily water consumption is the child's body weight divided by two. So if your child weighs 30 pounds, then they should be drinking at least 15 ounces of water each day.

Water-rich foods such as **fruits and vegetables** are essential to regular bowel movements. Not only are fruits and vegetables a great water source, but they are full of fiber as well. If you have a picky eater on your hands, you can get creative and hide them in your meals. Put spinach and kale in with apples, and they will not know the difference. You can also puree vegetables and put them in tomato sauce for pizza or pasta; they will not even know the difference. Also, encourage them to eat carrot or celery sticks with almond butter and raisins. You can even try to sneak some chia seeds into smoothies or anything else that you would puree.

Exercise is crucial to getting the bowels moving. The more you exercise, the more regular the bowels become. Exercise will also help you drink more fluids. Aerobic exercise, such as walking or running, will help to stimulate the bowel, as it increases the heart rate, in turn increasing blood flow so less water is absorbed, which allows your child to go to the bathroom. Make sure your children are involved in some sort of physical activity every day. Simple walking 20-30 minutes a day will aid in regular bowels. Doing jumping jacks, running in place, or even jumping up and down in place can make a difference.

Massage is always great to help relax the body and improve circulation. Babies love to be touched and massaging their belly and low back can help get the bowels moving. Massage is not just for adults; children need it as well. You can take baby massage classes to learn how to do it yourself, or have someone who is specially trained in babies to do the massage for you. When having a massage therapist work on your child, make sure they love kids and are comfortable working on children. Some have special training, but others do not, or do not feel comfortable working on children. It may take you a while to find someone you are comfortable with.

Sitting and playing video games, watching television, or sitting during school can cause things to slow down. These situations can be stressful, triggering the sympathetic nervous system (discussed more in-depth in Headache chapter), and slowing digestion and allowing more water to be absorbed into the stool, creating hard, and likely painful, stools. Practicing relaxation techniques like yoga and deep breathing will help to **lessen stress**.

Quick Reference for Constipation

1. Probiotics

2. Aloe Juice

3. Magnesium

4. Digestive Enzymes

5. Ileocecal Valve

6. Water

7. Omega 3's

8. Vitamin D

9. Massage

10. Fruits and Veggies

11. Exercise

12. Chiropractic Care

13. De-Stress

CHAPTER 4

WHY DIDN'T MY PEDIATRICIAN TELL ME ABOUT OTHER OPTIONS FOR REFLUX?

Second only to ear infections, reflux is one of the top reasons that parents choose to bring their children to my practice. Frequent spitting up, not sleeping, painful cries, arching of their back, and even crying without spit up (dubbed "silent reflux" by pediatricians), are all signs of a potential reflux issue.

Pediatricians' usually first recommend breastfeeding moms remove dairy from their diet. Formula feeding parents are told to try different formulas to find one that works for their baby, often coming up empty handed.

When dietary changes don't work, doctors begin prescribing H2 Histamine Blockers or acid reducers. They are a multi-billion dollar industry. The side effects of these medications include: headache, tiredness, dizziness, loss of appetite, upset stomach, vomiting, and diarrhea.

There have been no studies conducted on children under the age of one to determine the safety and efficacy of H2 Blockers. Some parents will notice that reflux has subsided from the calming of the stomach acid, but it isn't entirely solving the problem, and the baby is still spitting up.

When H2 Blockers fail, they move on to

something stronger, proton pump inhibitors (PPIs). These also decrease acid in the stomach by up to 90%. The effects and safety of these have not been studied on children either.

The problem with both H2 and PPI blockers is that they interfere with breaking down foods and can limit vitamin absorption such as B12, magnesium, iron, and calcium. (84) Further studies need to be done, but, you need to have stomach acid for digestion. If you are blocking acid, you are not breaking down foods as easily, and you can then become constipated and that leads to a new set of problems and medications.

Then while the body is nutrient poor from not breaking down foods, a new set of misguided medications is offered to help your child to go to the bathroom. This is a vicious cycle and can lead to many problems as the child age into adulthood. This contributes to today's epidemic of leaky gut and autoimmunity issues (see Headache Chapter for more information).

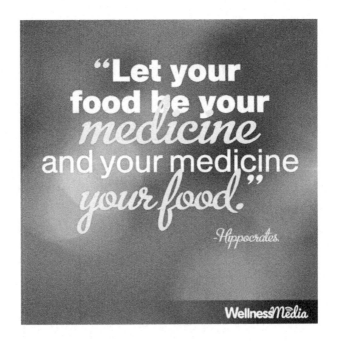

What can you do to naturally help stop the cycle of reflux? Here's the catch: *Did you know that reflux is actually caused by TOO LITTLE stomach acid?* It starts during pregnancy, as mom experiences heartburn and morning sickness, which can be carried to baby in-utero. If mom took an H2 or PPI during pregnancy, it can affect the baby as well.

As we get older, our acid levels drop, and we see an increase of GERD (gastroesophageal reflux disease).

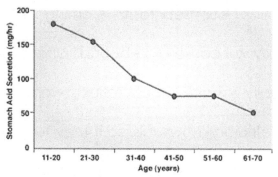

Fig. 1. Contrary to popular belief, stomach acid secretions drop with advancing age. This graph shows average decline in stomach acid secretion in humans between age 20 to age 80. (From "*Why Stomach Acid is Good For You.*")

These common medications are actually making the problem worse by suppressing the acid even more. The acid missing is called hydrochloric acid, or HCL. When HCL is low, an organism called Helicobacter pylori, or H. Pylori, causes a low-grade inflammation of the stomach lining, and the body's response is to want to get rid of it with reflux.

When coming off of these medications, it is important not to do so cold turkey. The body actually gets used to it. Coming off of it too quickly will cause a "rebound" effect, and can actually make the reflux worse. Your pediatrician knows this, so if they tell you to just stop, please don't. Take your time and try to work with your pediatrician.

Breastfeeding Moms

When a breastfed infant comes in with reflux issues, I need to find out about mom's diet, and anything that she is supplementing with. I also ask how her diet was during pregnancy, if she had heartburn, and if she used any medication or antibiotics to treat her symptoms. Often I have the mom supplement and change her diet before we do anything with the baby to keep their gut "virgin."

More than likely mom is deficient in **Vitamin D** since most OBGYN's do not test for it. If mom is a patient, then I test her levels. If not, then we supplement about 5,000 IUs of liquid vitamin D, as recommended by the Vitamin D Council. I usually recommend Xymogen brand. If you are not as concerned with keeping your child's gut "virgin", then you can supplement your child with 1,000 IU's per day.

I love **Probiotics**! They are amazing!! They help heal the gut and boost immunity. Did you know 85% of immunity comes from your gut? Your gut is considered like your second brain (more detail in the Headache chapter)(15) (16). The best way to get probiotics is to supplement. I like to have a broad spectrum of "good" bacteria. So you want to look for something with a minimum of 7-10 strain.

You don't just want to take acidophilus. Lactobacillus acidophilus is fortified in everything from bread, yogurt, milk, and cereals, so you can tend to get an overgrowth. I have seen kids break out, get rashes, and have dry or flaking skin from this.

In the office, we recommend Davinci Mega Probiotic or Klaire bland. They are vegetarian, gluten free, dairy free, and non-GMO. Wonderful products and we get great results with children and adults alike. Just remember, more doesn't always mean better. Follow the directions on any of the products you are using.

If you are interested in food source of probiotics, you can do kefir (like a liquid yogurt) or Kombucha. Both of these sources provide probiotics and support digestion health. You can get in the store or make your own if you have the time.

Mom can also incorporate **Digestive enzymes** along with probiotics. The enzymes will help break down fats, proteins, carbohydrates and milk sugars. Our foods today are not broken down like they once were due to being more processed. We need to help the body break down the food so it just doesn't sit in our stomach and intestines.

Mom's diet needs to be caffeine- and alcohol-free. It is also important to **limit dairy**, which produces histamines that cause irritation of the gut lining, decreasing the production of acid. (17)

I also recommend eliminating gluten/wheat from the diet as well. It can be difficult, and it takes longer for the body to completely rid itself of gluten. Eat as much organic as possible, including fruits and vegetables, as well as all organic meat and dairy (if you choose not to eliminate).

For meats and dairy, look for free-range, as well as antibiotic- and hormone-free. You may want to consider trying raw milk, if your state allows it, or goat's milk, as it is less inflammatory and closer to human's milk than cow's milk. (18).

Make sure you are drinking plenty of **water** to maintain your breast milk supply, and to keep your baby hydrated, as well.

Sea salt and **Himalayan Salt** will help the body to produce HCL (hydrochloric acid) in the stomach. For best results, be sure to choose an unrefined salt, not an iodized one. HCL actively fights off parasites and aids in digestion. This is where you can get your trace minerals. You can add to foods, or you can add a little to your water a few times a day. I personally add mine to my smoothies, I hardly know it is even in there.

Minerals are something we are often completely lacking in our diet. On average, we should be taking in approximately 80 essential minerals per day. Usually, we are lucky to get even 10-15 minerals on any given day, and diets rich in meat and processed foods can demineralize our bodies. (19) If you chose to ingest the sea salt, you will be getting minerals as well, but not everyone likes to add salt to their diet.

A great option would be to supplement with a **mineral complex**. Good mineral complex supplements should have between 60-80 different minerals. I recommend Youngevity's Cheri-Mins (http://youngevity.com/), which is one of the better ones I have found. You can find something similar to this at any vitamin shop. Please note, you will see trace amounts of metals and arsenic listed as ingredients on the bottle. These are all minerals that your body needs to flourish. Don't panic! Trust me, it is okay!

Lastly, my favorite is **aloe juice.** If you have not ever tried it, you are missing out. Aloe is amazing for digestive health (20), and especially for anyone struggling with reflux or constipation. Basically, the aloe goes in and coats the lining of the gut to allow it to heal from the repeated acidity that has irritated the lining so that nutrients can be absorbed.

You know how you use aloe to sooth a sunburn? This is the same concept; only it is the lining of the stomach and intestines. You will be pleased with the results! I recommend you get a flavored kind. Aloe by itself is a little bitter.

One downside with the flavored kinds is that it is often high sugar or artificially sweetened. So you may have to play around with different brands. Aloe is a more temporary measure to help break the cycle, and I feel the benefits can outweigh the downsides of sugars and sweeteners for a short amount of time.

Mom should drink 4oz in the morning on empty stomach and 4oz before night time on an empty stomach for 4-6 weeks or until the reflux has resolved. Having mom drink the aloe is another way to help soothe a baby's reflux while keeping the gut "virgin". You can find aloe at most health stores and chain stores. It is hiding in the laxative section. I have been recommending it for years, and not one person said they had loose bowels. In fact, they were going more regularly and happy with the results.

If you prefer, you can give the aloe directly to the baby, many parents prefer this method and feel they see better results. Dosing is listed below.

Non-Breastfed Babies

When integrating these techniques into a formula-fed baby's routine, much of what we just talked about above will be the same, except that the child will be getting the supplements directly rather than through their mother's milk.

Vitamin D can either be given by mouth or put in their bottle (1,000 IU's per day). Probiotics can be added to a prepared bottle of formula. You can either get a children's version, or if you have an adult version, you can open the capsule and empty its contents into a container. Then, take your finger, dip it in water, then in the probiotic, and swab their mouth with it.

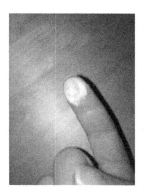

Or if you like, you can add about ¼ capsule to their bottle. Whichever method you choose, do this once per day. For the mineral complex, you can look for a children's version and follow the directions, or use an adult version and cut the dosage way back (no more than 1ml per day). You can even add a trace amount of salt to their bottle.

Aloe juice dosage varies depending on the size of the child, so you may have to try a few different amounts. Start small at first, and increase the dosage if you don't notice an improvement. If it seems like bowels are too loose, cut back.

Aloe amounts given 2 times a day (morning and night):

Infants 0-5 months	1-2 mL
6 months to 1 year	3-5 mL
Toddlers up to Age 5	1-2 ounces
6 - 10 years	2 ounces
11 - 13 years	3 ounces
14 - Adult	4 ounces

Toddlers to Young Adults

By the time I see toddlers or teenagers in my office for reflux or heartburn, they have been on medications for years. Transitioning children off of their medicines is not easy, and often they can get worse before they get better. Again, most of these medications decrease the acid of the stomach, but many children are already low in acid to begin with.

I always start with dietary changes: removing dairy and gluten product, increasing water intake, and supplementing with probiotics and digestive enzymes along with aloe juice to help soothe the lining and allow the probiotics to take over.

If need be, we may test for H. pylori, which is a bacteria that can cause ulcers. Many of us have this, and it does not cause any problems, but it may be a problem for others. In rare cases, I have had to supplement with HCL to help increase the acid production in the body.

I try not to do this, though, because I want the body to make its own acid. Changing the diet and adding probiotics will usually help to solve the problem, in addition to getting chiropractic care and working the trigger points, which we will be talking about more next.

The next best-kept secret is a trigger point for the **cardiac sphincter**. This is the junction where the esophagus and the stomach meet. It is a valve that controls what goes in and what comes out of the stomach including food and acid.

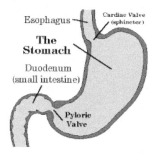

The sphincter can get stuck open from inflammation, so we want to help close the valve. The valve can be found just below the breastbone and the xyphoid process (the small knob below the main breastbone called the sternum).

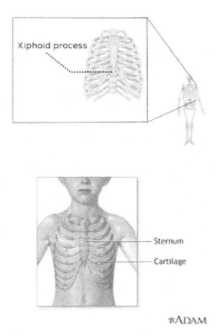

*ADAM

Once you find the knob, go just below it and you will feel a pocket of tissue without bone. That is where the sphincter is. Depending if the child is infant or older, you may use 1 or 2 fingers. Press down about ¼ to ½ inches. Aim your hand toward the feet almost like a scooping motion but use sustained pressure for 20-30 seconds after every feeding.

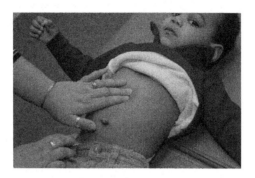

The first few times or days you do this, your child may be upset, cry, or push you away. This is all completely normal. They are telling you it's sore and inflamed. After doing this for over a period of days to weeks, depending how bad the reflux is, your child will start to calm down and enjoy it. Usually accompanying it is less reflux and a happier kid. Once you start seeing a decrease, then you can do it as needed.

Many kids with reflux also have constipation, and you may need to check the ileocecal valve as explained in the constipation chapter too.

Many parents like to put their baby in an upright position during the night, or some keep their kids in the car seat to help with the reflux. I do not recommend either of these things. The car seat can actually make the reflux worse by putting pressure on the abdomen and forcing foods or milk back up.

The best way to keep a baby upright is at a **slight angle**. You can use a wedge or a small towel under the baby to prop them up slightly. This will keep baby at only a slight incline while still keeping their body in alignment for proper digestion. In the day time, wearing your baby will also help with keeping upright for reflux.

Once again, **chiropractic care** can help with relieving reflux. Misalignments from the upper neck due to childbirth or improper positioning in the womb can be a major cause of spitting up. I see it often with breech babies and doctor-assisted births where the baby's head is pulled or suctioned by the OBGYN to get the baby out of the canal.

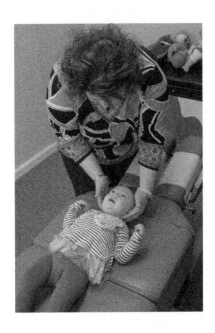

There can be 90-140 pounds of pressure on the baby's head and body during delivery (85). That would be about the same as 2,000 pounds exerted on a 200 pound man. Also, some babies are delivered with forceps or a vacuum which can cause birth trauma, such as shoulder dystocia, torticollis, and skull deformities which I see and feel on a daily basis. Enormous force may have been exerted on the baby's head and neck. Because of this, it is a great idea to have every newborn checked by a chiropractic physician who specializes in pediatric care.

You will notice many babies with reflux and other related issues arch their back, look uncomfortable, or cry a lot. Many times colic and reflux go hand in hand. Arching is not normal. Regular chiropractic adjustments will help to calm the muscles down and align the spine to allow the body to function effectively.

Quick Reference for Reflux:

1. Aloe Juice

2. Vitamin D

3. Probiotics/digestive enzymes

4. Do not come off medicines abruptly

5. Cardiac Sphincter

6. Chiropractic Care

CHAPTER 5

WHY DIDN'T MY PEDIATRICIAN TELL ME ABOUT THE DIFFERENCE BETWEEN AN EAR INFECTION AND TEETHING?

It's 2 o'clock in the morning and you are sound asleep when a horror movie-worthy scream comes from your child's bedroom. They are frantic, screaming, and pulling on their ear. Your heart is pounding, and you are not sure what to do. Has this happened to you? I hear this story all the time in the office. These are classic signs of an ear infection or Otitis Media. Or is your child teething?

With over 10 million cases per year and rising, ear

infections and ear aches are the number one reason for pediatric visits, as well as one of the most misdiagnosed. The standard care of practice for pediatricians (even though the American Academy of Pediatrics has called for a more wait-and-see approach) is antibiotics, usually without even knowing if the infections are bacterial in nature. Then, when the first round doesn't work, more antibiotics are prescribed, then an even stronger one, and now you are in the never ending antibiotic and ear infection cycle.

Your frustration is building, and your child is not getting any better. If the first two or three rounds of antibiotics have failed, why do they keep prescribing antibiotics? Maybe the ear infection is viral, so the antibiotic will not work. Or are our babies just teething?

Teething can mimic an ear infection very easily. Kids are drooling, gums are swollen, have a runny nose and fever, and are just not feeling well. Remember the ears, nose, mouth, throat, and neck are all connected. As the gums begin to swell, they become inflamed which leads to swelling of the upper neck and ears. This can cause the ears to look pink or red, and may cause pain. Many children develop a rash on their face or on their buttocks called the "teething rash."

Usually, there is not an infection, but since the ears look red or pink and babies are uncomfortable and tugging at their ears, it is typically treated as an infection. Sometimes when the ears are swollen, there is fluid in the ears because it can't drain. Once the swelling is down, the fluid will disappear. It can take up to 2 years for baby teeth to come in completely, with the molars usually taking the longest. They are the teeth closest to the ears, so the confusion of symptoms is very common.

Since none of the antibiotics have worked, they are now considering ear tubes. Guess what? <u>The number one complication of tubes is that the ear infections will not go away</u>. Your child may experience hearing loss, constant drainage, a hole made of scar tissue from repeated tubes with green or yellow drainage all day and night, or need further and more aggressive surgery such as tonsil, adenoid, sinus, or ear surgery. Adenoid surgery is now becoming very common in children with failed tubes, and I am seeing it in my office more than I should. Ear tubes are the number ONE outpatient surgery for children, and 25% of children will get repeated tubes. "You've got the number-one ambulatory surgery in kids, the number-one reason they are given anesthesia, and no national society has ever published evidence-based guidelines about the best way to do this," said Dr. Richard Rosenfeld, a professor and chairman of otolaryngology at SUNY Downstate Medical Center in Brooklyn, New York.

The result of 41 studies found there was a

temporary increase in hearing with tubes, but no difference in language, cognitive, or academic outcomes.

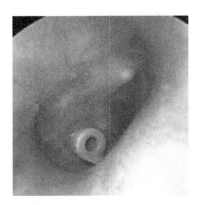

If your child happens to have a fever with the ear ache, DO NOT suppress it! If it is a low-grade fever (100-102 degrees), let your child ride it out. Fever is a natural way for the body to rid itself of viruses. By suppressing the fever, you can actually make the infection last longer. Did you know teething causes fever too?

Did your pediatrician tell you about any side effects of antibiotics? Some side effects include nausea, vomiting, diarrhea, abdominal pain, yeast and candida, and antibiotics can lead to leaky gut which will be explained more in depth in a later chapter. Dr. J. Owen Hendley, a Pediatrician from the University of Virginia, reviewed 100 studies on antibiotics and their effects of antibiotics and otitis media and found <u>ONLY 1 in 8 actually helped children </u>(21).

That's only a 12.5% chance of helping your child's ear infections. Keep in mind that over 60% of ear aches will go away on their own without any antibiotics whatsoever within 3 months.

The biggest thing to remember is that antibiotics

do not discriminate between a good bacteria and a bad bacteria. So, if the good bacteria is not repopulated with a probiotic, you are possibly potentially setting your child up for more infections, constipation, and more frequent cases of the cold and flu. Your probiotic should be a broad spectrum supplement, with 7-10 different healthy bacteria not just Lactobacillus acidophilus that which is found in yogurt. A healthy child has a healthy gut!

Surveys show that unvaccinated children are generally healthier and experience fewer colds and flus than their vaccinated counterparts. A survey from New Zealand found vaccinated children were 3 times as likely to get ear infections than those who had not been vaccinated. A survey in Germany of over 7,866 children found Otitis Media to be doubled in vaccinated children. The latest and ongoing survey by Vaccinelnjury.info has over 7,850 entries so far, and has found vaccinated children have 22 times the ear infections than those who are not vaccinated. This is a worldwide survey not looking at one particular area.

Many parents are now looking for a more natural way of dealing with otitis media and teething, as they are tired of giving their children medications without seeing results. In addition to **probiotics,** I recommend **_liquid_ Vitamin D**. Both the probiotics and the Vitamin D will help boost and support your child's immune system. I have lab tested patients who have taken 8 weeks of liquid gels, then had them take 8 weeks of liquid, and unlike the gel caps, the liquid supplement brought their levels within the 60-80ng/ml range. Over 32% of children and adults are Vitamin D deficient according to the Center for Disease Control and Prevention.

The National Health and Nutrition Examination Survey found that 50 percent of children aged 1 to 5 years old, and 70 percent of children between the ages of 6 and 11, are low in Vitamin D. Mom should be taking Vitamin D during pregnancy to help babies in the long run. According to the Vitamin D Council, Vitamin D does pass through breast milk.

Amber necklaces may help teething and ear

aches. Beware, there are many out there that are not pure amber, so look for a good one and spend a little money. Make sure each stone is wrapped individually to prevent a choking hazard in case they break. I have been carrying them for several years and I have not had one returned from being broken.

While worn, the skin heats up the amber and then it releases an oil which can allow microscopic amounts to absorb into the bloodstream and help to calm a fussy child.

It can help reduce swelling of the gums and ears, and many say they see an improvement of the infections as well as notice less complaining of ears hurting. Many parents ask me, "How do I know if the necklace is working?" My response is to take it off for a few days and see what happens. They usually have the necklace back on within a few hours.

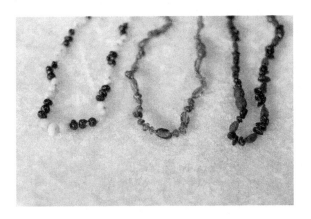

What else can you do to help your child from all the tugging and complaining? You can **remove dairy** from their diet until the pain has subsided. Dairy is considered very inflammatory and can cause mucous buildup. The sugars and protein in milk are acidic, and many children are allergic and don't even know it. Casein found in milk is the second most inflammatory food, only behind gluten.

They have a similar structure, so many people with gluten sensitivity are also casein sensitive. You can get calcium from many other sources like almonds, spinach, kale, and oranges. Rest assured, if you cut out dairy, your child will not go without. Many children also have sensitivity to soy, corn, processed foods with sugars, and peanuts, so further allergy testing may be needed to get to the bottom of inflammation and Otitis Media.

There are so many different things you can put in your child's ear to help sooth them. If you are nursing, put a little breast milk in their ears. 3-4 drops will do. **Breast milk** is full of antibodies, so it provides many health benefits! You can also use **Colloidal Silver** (this should be in your house at all times). It is amazing! It is a natural antibiotic, antiseptic, and antifungal. Not only is it wonderful for ear infections, but also cuts, scrapes, colds, and flu.

For ears, put 1-2 drops in the ear in the morning and at night. Your child can also ingest small amounts to help fight off any high fevers associated with the infection or teething.

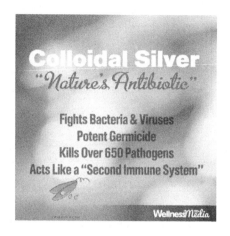

When you are doing your research, you will find like that most natural remedies are not FDA approved, which is the stock answer you'll get from most pediatricians. My response to that is, according to the FDA: *"Singh [2000] estimated that 103,000 individuals are hospitalized annually in the United States for NSAID-related serious gastrointestinal complications at a cost in excess of two billion dollars. In addition, Singh [2000] estimated that 16,500 NSAID-related deaths*

occur each year in the United States among patients with rheumatoid arthritis and osteoarthritis.

Presumably, these estimates are based primarily on prescription NSAIDs used for longer time periods than the OTC label recommends, but as noted earlier, some individuals may use OTC NSAIDs in excess of the OTC recommended dose or take two or more OTC NSAIDs concurrently."(67)

NSAIDs are FDA approved, and 103,000 hospitalizations for GI bleeds annually back in 2000 (I'm sure that number today is much higher). That is not acceptable. Doing my research, I could not find one death or hospitalization from someone using colloidal silver or aloe juice.

Tea Tree Oil (Melaleuca Oil) is wonderful, as well. Tea tree is known for its soothing, antiseptic and antimicrobial properties. The oil is great for ear infections, and many people use it on acne, their scalp, and help to rid hair of lice. We also use it on burns, on skin, or cuts and scrapes, too. Make sure it is out of reach, as it is toxic and not safe to ingest. Some of our parents in the office like to use **Garlic Oil.**

You can make your own by putting a few cloves of garlic on some olive oil, and let sit overnight. Then you can add 1-2 drops in the ear each day. Make sure you remove the garlic from the bottle of oil, and you can use the garlic in the future for cooking. You want to make sure no garlic pieces enter your child's ear. This is not my favorite method of soothing ears, but many moms have great luck with it, and it is a less expensive route than some of the other oils.

Ever hear of the **Magic Salt Sock**? This little trick is amazing! A fellow chiropractor came up with the idea, and it can really help with relieving the pain.(86) You will need a white sock (it CANNOT be colored), and 1 cup of COARSE SEA SALT (it has to be sea salt and it has to be coarse, or it will seep through the sock. Fill the sock with the salt, then put it in the microwave starting at 30 second increments (since every microwave is different). If you do not have a microwave, wrap it in foil and use a pan on low to warm the sock, turning it every 30-60 seconds. Make sure you shake the sock with every turn to make sure the heat is distributed evenly. The sock should be warm, but not so hot that you cannot touch the skin.

If your child will lay down, have them lay the problem ear down on top of the Magic Salt Sock, and let them relax for a while. You can always sit if it is too painful to lay down. The salty air will help to dry out the infection or fluid that is in the ear and help ease the pain. You can reuse the sock until the sock starts to get discolored or starts to fall apart. You will be amazed at how well it works!

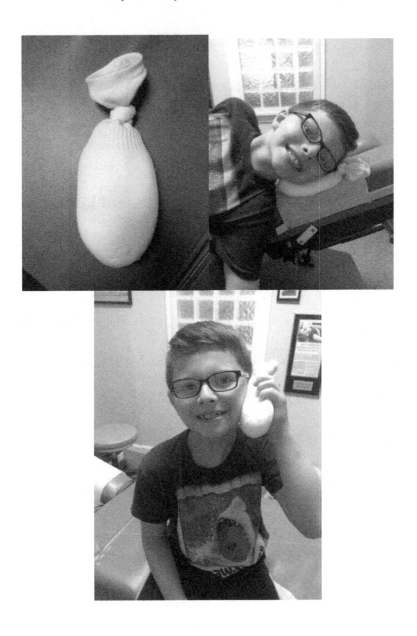

If your doctor has said there is a lot of wax in your

child's ear and they have tried to clean it out with no luck, you may want to try **ear candling**. It is a non-invasive way to clean ears. I would not recommend you do this at home, but rather at have a professional do this. Many massage and integrative practices will do this in their offices.

Ear candling helps to soften up the wax buildup to make it easier to get rid of it. As the candle burns, your child will feel warmth and at times hear sizzling; that is the wax getting warm. It doesn't hurt them, it's just warmth. After the candle is done, you can open it up and see what is in the candle. There will be parts that look like wax, but it isn't all from your child's ear, some are the candle itself. Many will say they feel something draining when done, which is good.

You may also want to try rinsing the ear with warm water after the candling. Many times you will see wax coming out since the candle broke it up a little. Many say they can hear and breathe better. The biggest most important thing is to make sure your child lays still during the candling. This isn't for everyone, but it is an option.

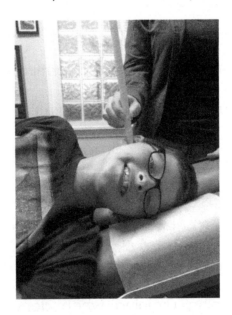

If your child is teething, there are a few things you can do. You can brew some **Chamomile tea** and soak a washcloth or a new clean sock in the tea and then freeze it. You can then let your child chew on it to help soothe the swollen gums. There are homeopathic **teething tablets** that many parents swear by.

They work great for those really bad nights when the pressure is building up in their gums and ears when they lay down. I usually recommend Hyland's brand tablets. There are other brands out there, but I get the best feedback from this product. www.hylands.com.

If you don't have **Sophie la giraffe** you are missing out! This is great for teething! It has long legs so it is wonderful to get the back molars. It is made from 100% natural rubber and is non-toxic. It also helps to encourage sight, smell, and touch.

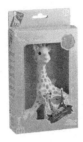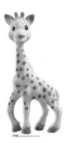

Many parents are surprised how well **chiropractic care** can help with ear infections and aches. Chiropractic care, as stated before, is very safe and gentle. When searching for a chiropractor in your area, make sure they are Board Certified in pediatrics through International Chiropractic Pediatric Association (ICPA) or International Chiropractors Association Council on Chiropractic Pediatrics. Both are wonderful post-doctorate programs, providing the skills and knowledge for us to be up to date on the most recent information and applications for naturally healing your child.

A study of 332 children suffering from otitis media, published in the Journal of Clinical Chiropractic Pediatrics, found ear infections were resolved after an average of 4 visits, with 5 visits for chronic cases. (22) Another study found a 93% improvement of ear infections within 10 days or fewer, and for 43% it only took 1-2 visits to help with otitis media. (23)

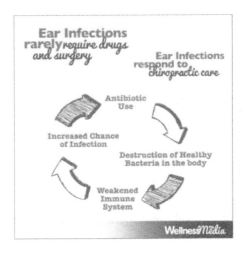

Chiropractic care helps to break the cycle, and the studies suggest adjustment can be more effective than drug therapy. The best part is that the adjustments are non-invasive and completely drug-free! Don't forget, the American Academy of Pediatrics' stance is to take the wait-and-see approach before giving antibiotics due to many people becoming antibiotic resistant, so chiropractic care and efforts to repopulate the gut with nutrients while you are waiting will help with resolving Otitis Media.

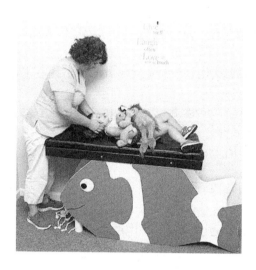

During an ear infection, I have parents **stop dairy** until we are in the clear. Dairy can be inflammatory and can cause a runny nose and clogged ears. If you want to see an even bigger improvement, remove gluten from their diet, as well, so they are dairy and gluten-free. You can do this for short times, like just during the episodes, or on a continuous basis.

I know that neither of these are particularly easy to cut out, so we have to pick our battles. I usually start with dairy, as that is the easier food group to remove from diets. Gluten is harder to do, as it is in many of our foods today. The good news is there are so many more options for gluten-free foods out there today. Make sure your children are eating plenty fruits and vegetables, and also drinking plenty of water.

Quick Reference for Ear Infections

1. Vitamin D and broad spectrum probiotic

2. Tea Tree Oil, garlic oil, breast milk, colloidal silver

3. Amber Teething Necklace

4. Chiropractic care

5. Magic Salt Sock

6. Wait and see approach

7. Remove dairy and gluten

CHAPTER 6

WHY DIDN'T MY PEDIATRICIAN TELL ME ABOUT OTHER OPTIONS FOR ASTHMA?

I'm sure many of you parents have heard the words, "There is NO CURE for asthma," or the ever-popular, "They will grow out of it." I know the parents who come to my office are told that all the time, and that is not an acceptable answer. Those of you that are looking for other options and are tired of all the medications and steroids, please know that the statement is not true.

Many have found diet changes very helpful in controlling asthma. Others have found that their child is allergic to something or discovered that adding supplements as simple as a good multivitamin have helped. Parents also see a world of difference with chiropractic care, and clinical trials and studies are looking promising.

What exactly is Asthma and what are the symptoms? According to the National Institute of Health, Asthma is a chronic and incurable lung disease that narrows and inflames the airway causing wheezing and coughing, tightness in the chest, and shortness of breath. As the airway narrows, and less air is moving through the lungs, cells can start to produce mucous making the airways even smaller.

The American Lung Association (ALA) states over

7.1 million children under 18 years of age suffer from the disease; 4.1 million of whom experienced an asthma attack or episode in 2011. Those are some staggering statistics. Asthma is second in childhood illness behind ear infections. Here's another wonderful statistic from the ALA: **"Asthma is one of the leading causes of school absenteeism**; in 2008, asthma accounted for an estimated 14.4 million lost school days in children with an asthma attack in the previous year."

All of these numbers are on the rise. Why are the numbers rising so much? We now have so many environmental toxins, food allergies, vaccines, processed foods, and genetically modified foods (GMO's) that we were not so exposed to in the past. Not to mention the rise of cesarean births in some states is at 33%, and the over-prescribing of antibiotics. Also, taking acetaminophen and ibuprofen during pregnancy, which is a common recommendation from OBGYN's, and giving it to your child at an early age can increase the risk of asthma.(68) So it is a good idea to skip the pain relievers if you can.

Vaccines can increase a child's risk of asthma, as well. Vaccines raise your T2 Helper cell count, which, during pregnancy, can cause your child to have an imbalance of their Th1/th2 ratio. The higher the T2 ratio, the more asthma, eczema, and autoimmunity disorders you child can have (9)(10). (See the wellness chapter for more vaccine information) Many times after a vaccine, children will get a fever; fever is your body's natural way to defend itself against a foreign substance or virus, and the pediatrician recommends to take some Tylenol or ibuprofen to decrease the fever, both can increase asthma. Does this make sense to you? Are we just setting our children up for asthma?

So, what can you do to avoid your child from becoming a statistic? When a child comes to my office with asthma or difficulty breathing, first and foremost, they **get aligned**! This is not an option in care at my office, and here is why: in the Journal of Orthopedic Surgery's study of 3,013 patients with Bronchial asthma published in 2004, they were able to "alleviate bronchial asthma and allergies by improvement of Neurology caused by chronically narrowed intervertebral foramina from the 2nd to the 4th and 8th to the 10th thoracic vertebrae...Asthma patients improved by 70%." What this means is that misalignments of the spine in the mid-back of your child can be causing the asthma symptoms. This is why chiropractic is SO important for the health of your child! (24)

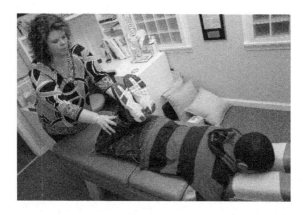

In another random clinical trial, 36 children with chronic pediatric asthma were studied over a 3-month period, along with medical care (25).

Those with chiropractic care had extremely improved quality care and decreased asthma severity, while those children under standard medical pulmonary treatments showed little to no statistical significance.

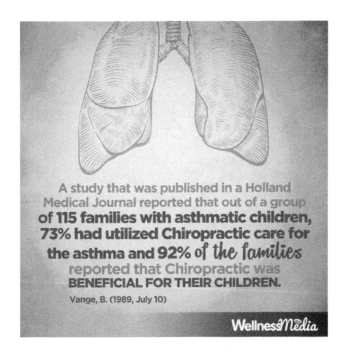

A study that was published in a Holland Medical Journal reported that out of a group of 115 families with asthmatic children, 73% had utilized Chiropractic care for the asthma and 92% of the families reported that Chiropractic was BENEFICIAL FOR THEIR CHILDREN.

Vange, B. (1989, July 10)

Wellness Media

Another study by the Journal of Vertebral Subluxation Research of 81 asthmatic children reported an improvement in 90.1% after being under chiropractic care for 60 days; ages ranged from 1-17 years of age. The number of asthma "attacks" decreased by an average of 44.9%, and 30.9% decreased their medication by 66.5%. The authors concluded that "Chiropractic care, for correction of vertebral subluxation, is a safe, non-pharmaceutical health care approach which may also be associated with significant decreases in asthma-related impairment as well as a decreased incidence of asthmatic `attacks.'"(26)

These studies are why chiropractic care is imperative to the health of your child who has been suffering with asthma. Once chiropractic care is underway, we start looking at diet and supplements. I usually will order lab work and look at different vitamins and minerals. I will usually look at thyroid, Vitamin D, calcium, iron, magnesium, B vitamins, IgG's of Gluten and Casein (baseline of milk and wheat allergy are the most common; but we may need to look further into other food allergies).

While we are waiting for all the labs to come back, I need to look at a food diary; everything that passes through your child's mouth, including drinks, will need to be recorded. This diary will also track how much sleep your child is getting a night, and how many and what kind of animals are in the house, the presence of cigarette smoke in the house, or if there is mold that could worsen the asthma. It is important to look in windows, pull out the dishwasher, (and) clean the vents of the house to help keep mold out. Many children with asthma do better without carpet in the house. Hardwood or concrete are cleaner and do not trap dust and dander, so cleaning and dusting are a top priority.

With over half of your body being comprised of water, make sure your child is drinking plenty of water; just **water** with nothing added. You may add a lemon or lime slice if you like, but, no added packets of sweeteners or things to make the water change color and add flavor. Just plain water. The rule of thumb for daily water intake is body weight (in pounds), divided by 2. That is how many ounces your child should drink. It takes a lot to stay hydrated, but it is so important.

Body Weight in Pounds/2= Water in Ounces

Just as water is important to the body, you must breathe. You can live 2-3 days without water, but you can only live 3 minutes without air. A child with asthma must do deep breathing exercises to get oxygen not only to the lungs, but also throughout the body for fuel. As a nation, we are oxygen deprived; we are over-stressed and in turn, we are shallow breathers.

As a family, you can do this at night: Slowly take in a long, deep breath in through your nose (holding to a count of 7), then exhale slowly through the mouth until there is no air left in the lungs. You will want to do this 3-4 times in one sitting. If you have the time, at least have your child do this before they go to school. They need the oxygen to fuel their brain, and if your child practices these breathing exercises regularly, you will see them sleep better, their digestion will improve, and of course, they will be breathing better.

Getting back to diet, it is important to examine the link between gluten, casein, and the gut. A child may not have Celiac Disease (an autoimmune disease that attacks the small intestine due to gluten), but rather, they may be gluten-sensitive.

For an asthmatic child, it is very important to remove or limit dairy because it is mucous-producing, and to limit or eliminate gluten because of the inflammation. **Dairy** products include milk, cheese, yogurt, ice cream, etc. **Gluten** products are grains (wheat, rye, barley). That means no pizza, pasta, bread, or crackers unless they are Certified Gluten Free. Watch out, though, many CGF products are full of sugars and are very processed, so you may want to skip these products altogether while your child is in the healing process.

I always advise when grocery shopping, to only walk around the perimeter. That is where all the whole foods are fruits and vegetables, meats, and dairy. Generally, nothing on the outside perimeter is processed. So, always avoid the aisles when purchasing foods, and go raw organic if it is in your budget.

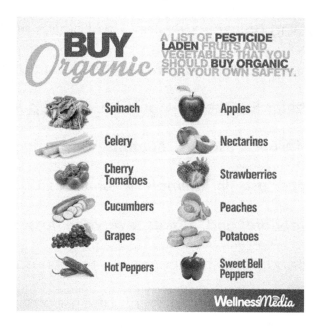

So, what is the best diet for an asthmatic child?

Paleo! Paleo is a diet full of fruits and vegetables,

and you do get protein from meats and fish, but

no grains at all. Animal protein must be grass-fed

(not grain-fed), free range, and especially

antibiotic- and hormone-free! Between the

antibiotics in our meats and the ones we are

over-prescribed as a nation, our bodies are becoming antibiotic resistant. Antibiotics are not working for us like they once were. According to the Center for Disease Control (CDC) *"Up to half of antibiotic use in humans and much of antibiotic use in animals is unnecessary and inappropriate and makes everyone less safe."* *(27)* Because of the increased hormones in the food, girls are hitting puberty at an earlier age, and we are also seeing an increase of breast and prostate cancer due to the increased estrogen and testosterone in cattle and sheep.

As far as supplementation goes, it all depends on what the lab work shows. The biggest deficiencies are generally in Vitamin D, magnesium, and iron. Some children can be hypothyroid, and that is why I do a full panel so we can supplement with desiccated thyroid products instead of medications, if needed.

As stated before, **Vitamin D** numbers should be around 60-80ng/ml. If Vitamin D numbers are in the 10-20 range, I would start on 5,000 IUs a day for 2 weeks, then drop to 2,000 IUs per day for 4 weeks, then recheck the numbers, all depending on the age of the child.

Magnesium is a common mineral we are all deficient in, not just children. This helps to calm and relax our body. This mineral is imperative for asthmatic children because their ribs and chest muscles get so tight. Depending on how low the labs are, I suggest anywhere from 500-1000mg of magnesium at night time. Taking it at night will help with sleep.

If your child is getting too much magnesium, it can cause loose stools or diarrhea, so that is something to watch out for. That is why I have them take the supplement at night, so they are home. If that happens, cut back about 100-200mg until their bowels are normal. This usually is not a problem, since many children are not having bowel movements 2-3 times a day as they should be. Magnesium will also help with becoming "regular", along with easing aches and pains, as well.

Omega 3's, or essential fatty acids (EFA), found in fish oils have an anti-inflammatory properties for the body. A study from the University of Sydney found children who eat oily fish on a regular basis are 4 times less likely to develop asthma than those children who do not eat fish. They are speculating that EFA's help in decreasing the severity of asthma due to reducing the inflammation in the airway. (28) Fish oil is comprised of two acids, eicosapentaenoic acid (EPA) and docosahexaenoic acid (DHA). You can get EFA through eating fresh, cold water fish 2-3 times a week, or you can supplement.

I recommend 1-3 grams of EPA + DHA together each day for children. Not only will it help decrease inflammation, but it will help with brain and heart development.

With our American diet, we consume a higher ratio (average 20 times) of Omega 6's than Omega 3's in our foods. These EFA are more inflammatory and are found in vegetable oils based from corn and soy oils, rather than fish. Because of our diet, this is why consuming Omega 3's are so important.

It is also important that your child is on a great broad spectrum **probiotic,** 7-10 strands, preferably dairy-free. Probiotics are great in aiding to heal the gut and helps to boost the immune system. Many of our children also benefit from **Juice Plus**. It is your fruits and vegetables all in one place. This helps many children who are picky about eating fruits and vegetables to have an alternative to help bridge the gap of what they are missing in their diet. You can go to their website, www.juiceplus.com, to learn more.

Essential Oils and asthma have been a controversial topic for some time. Many have said the smells can trigger an attack while many say some can help. In the office, we tend to play it safe. We mainly use <u>Lavender</u> and <u>Frankincense</u> for asthmatics. Both of these oils have anti-inflammatory properties to them to help open up the lungs.

You can use the oils several ways: you can diffuse them by adding 2-8 drops each in a diffuser for the room, or you can apply on the chest as a rub. Add 2-4 drops of each to a carrier oil (we recommend coconut oil) and rub over the chest area of your child. This way it can be absorbed in the body to help fight inflammation.

If you or your child do not like the smell of the oils, you can place a few drops on their feet and then cover with a sock. Feet are not only wonderful for absorption, but also great in helping to stimulate the brain. That is why barefoot is best (we will talk about that more in the posture chapter).

Don't forget to get your child out to **exercise**. Walking, swimming, and bike riding are all great! Yoga is also a great way to help open up the lungs and expand the chest and the muscles surrounding the ribcage. These exercises tend to be low impact, so they shouldn't affect their breathing too much. As your child heals, they can start to do more vigorous exercising.

As you can see, there are many things you can do to help with your child's asthma. I know it can be scary, especially during attacks, but I know many of these alternative remedies are helping so many children in my office!

Quick Reference for Asthma

1. Chiropractic Care

2. Paleo Diet—Gluten and Dairy Free

3. Water

4. Vitamin D, Probiotics

5. Omega 3's

6. Magnesium

7. Essential Oils- Lavender and Frankincense

8. Exercise

CHAPTER 7

WHY DIDN'T MY PEDIATRICIAN TELL ME ABOUT HELPING MY CHILD WITH HEADACHES?

UGGGGHHH, headaches. As an adult, you know how much a headache can affect your life. They make it hard to see, impossible to concentrate, and difficult to think straight. Let's face it, headaches are not fun and can be debilitating.

Many adults that suffer with migraines today say that they had headaches growing up as a child, so as a practitioner, I need to stop the headaches at an early age to help my patients as they transition into adulthood. I cannot tell you how frustrated I get by the commercials touting daily headaches. ***Daily Headaches Are Not Normal!*** There is a reason why your child is getting headaches, and we need to get to the bottom of it.

75% of children will get headaches before the age of 15, with girls being more affected than boys. That is quite a staggering number, and the numbers are of course rising due to our American lifestyle. (29)

According to the National Headache Foundation, the most common headache in children is a **tension headache**, sometimes called **cervicogenic**, or what I like to call **text neck**.

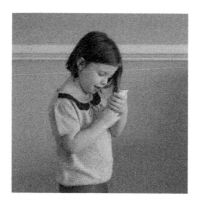

The main cause of these types of headaches is Poor Posture from looking down for long periods of time.   Posture will be discussed in an <u>entire</u> chapter later in the book because posture is THAT important. Tension headaches start in the neck and can wrap around the head.

Many children in my office also complain of neck and shoulder pain or tightness in addition to their headaches. Their muscles are usually hot and extremely tight, and patients typically have a limited range of motion in their neck. Below is a typical child at school, doing work. Looking at the rounded shoulders and the strain on their neck, it's no wonder children's tension headaches are on the rise. Using a book stand can help raise up the neck and release the tension in the muscles from overuse.

If you look at the children texting, the girl's head in the picture above is not even over her shoulders, causing forward head posture up to an extra 10-20 pounds of pressure being exerted on the neck. I'm sure if you look at your children you will see similar posture while they are texting.

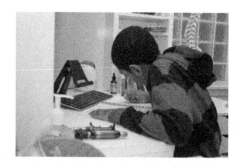

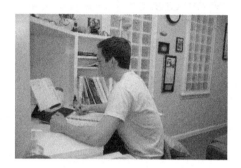

Another type of headache common to children

is the classic **Migraine Headache,** or **vascular**

headache. Symptoms include sensitivity to light,

sound, and touch, nausea, seeing auras, lack of

energy, dizziness, and sleepiness. Migraine

headaches stem from the autonomic nervous

system (ANS) and has been termed "sympathetic

nervous system dysfunction". (30)

The easiest way to explain the autonomic nervous system or ANS is to divide it into 3 parts: sympathetic, parasympathetic, and enteric systems. Why are all three of these symptoms important to your child? The ANS controls muscle, gland, and organ function.

The Sympathetic is triggered during stressful times, termed "fight or flight." It increases your heart rate, constricts blood vessels, raises your blood pressure, and slows down digestion. The Parasympathetic is your "rest and digest" system. It increases digestion and relaxes muscles, lowers the heart rate, and increases gland secretions.

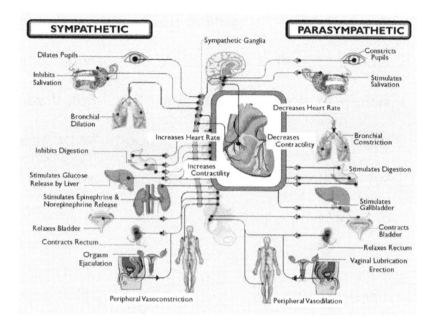

Lastly, the enteric system is a mesh-like system of neurons surrounding the gastrointestinal (GI) tract and is considered your "second brain". It can function on its own, or work with the parasympathetic and/or sympathetic systems together. The main purpose is to help aid in digestion, to expel waste, and to aid in nutrient absorption. This system is the most complex.

The tricky part is getting all the symptoms to function together evenly. We do not want one system to dominate over the other. But, if you pay close attention to the sympathetic picture, you will notice most child and adults are in fight or flight/ sympathetic mode.

For example:

- Inhibits digestion=constipation or heartburn/reflux
- Inhibits salvation= dry mouth
- Stimulates Glucose to be released= high blood sugar or diabetes
- Relaxes bladder= bedwetting or incontinence
- Dilates Pupils= light sensitivity—like to wear sunglasses even indoors.

So, why did I take all this time to go through the nervous system? It is important to realize how important the system is, and how much it controls your entire body. **<u>Chiropractic care has been found to be very beneficial in helping with headaches and balances all three nervous systems.</u>**

A study from 2001 found chiropractic care resulted in immediate improvement in headache severity when used to treat episodes of cervicogenic headache when compared with an attention-placebo control. (31)

In another study of 127 participants complaining of migraines, patients underwent chiropractic treatments to see if it would help. Ages ranged from 10-70, and over 80% of them reported being high-stress. 22% of participants reported a 90% reduction in their migraines while another 50% reported significant improvement in the morbidity of each episode.

The study concluded by saying: *"It appears probable that chiropractic care has an effect on the physical conditions related to stress and that in these people the effects of the migraine are reduced."* (32) Children are now under more stress and demands than ever before. Between the stress of academic performance and behavior expectations in school, to extracurricular activities like sports or band, to caring for a younger sibling after school, in addition to poor posture and a generally poor diet, the perfect storm is brewing for headaches.

As you can see, it is important to have regular chiropractic adjustments not only for adults but children too. This will help to balance the nervous system in our overstressed lives. Once again, you can find a pediatric chiropractor through International Chiropractic Pediatric Association. www.icpa4kids.org

Don't forget to try to do some **light exercise**, even if it is just walking. Doing exercise will help improve circulation to the entire body. The blood will help to get nutrients and oxygen to the body and the brain. Exercise also will help to decrease stress not only mentally, but physically, as well. The increase in exercise will aid in digestion and help with improved sleep as well.

Diet is very important when dealing with headaches. Make sure your children are hydrated with water first and foremost. Oftentimes, water is not allowed in classrooms, and I actually have to write my patients a note saying that they are allowed water in the classroom. Don't be afraid to ask your physician for a note for your child.

Do not skip breakfast! It is so important so to fuel the brain and body at the start of the day. The meal should not be too heavy, but a smoothie is the perfect way to get in fruits and vegetables, and will sustain your child through the morning more so than a box of sugary cereal. I also recommend for your child to have snacks during the school day, too. This will help to maintain an appropriate blood sugar and help to keep your child awake and alert for school.

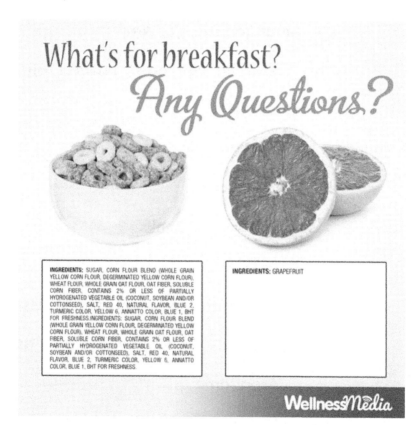

Good Snacks

- **Nuts**

- **Fruits**

- **Vegetables**

- **Protein Drink or Smoothie**

- **Small Sandwich or Wrap**

- **Protein or Fruit bars. (Quest and Larabars)**

Poor Snacks and Headache Triggers:

- **Chocolate**

- **Caffeinated Drinks**

- **Dairy**

- **Processed Foods, including Meats**

- **Artificial Sweeteners such as Aspartame**

- **Gluten or Wheat**

- **Monosodium Glutamate (MSG)**

I have many families keep a **Headache Log**, tracking what their child eats, how much they sleep, their daily activities, and if they were feeling stressed so we can find out if there is a pattern. The above snack list is not a complete list by any means, and your son or daughter may have a trigger that is not on the list. Further food allergy testing may have to be done to pinpoint the exact allergen.

There is a new headache on the rise. It is termed the **New Daily Persistent Headache.** This type of headache is not yet completely understood, but in dealing with patients on a clinical basis, we have determined that it can be biochemical, possibly hormonal. Once again, _daily headaches are not normal_, so let's start looking at thyroid, Vitamin D, and adrenal glands and their effect on headaches.

The **thyroid** in children is often overlooked. Many pediatricians tend to dismiss the thyroid altogether. A full thyroid panel of lab work is not often done in children, but should be done more often. Make sure they are looking at not only TSH and Free T4, but also Free T3 and Total T3 and T4.

What exactly is the thyroid? It is a butterfly-shaped gland that is in the neck, just below your Adam's apple. It aids in brain development in children, secretes hormones, regulates your temperature, and helps in metabolism. This gland is very important, so why is it not being checked more often?

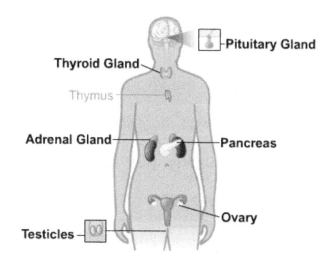

National Institutes of Health U.S. National Library of Medicine

Just like your thyroid, **Vitamin D**, or the sunshine vitamin, is extremely important to your body. Vitamin D is best supplemented with the sun, which is how it gets its name. 85% of the United States population are deficient and don't even know it. I'm often asked, "I drink milk so I should be getting enough in that, right?" Wrong. Many companies are "fortifying" Vitamin D into milk, yogurt, and cereal, usually around 100-400 IU's, and it simply isn't enough. Here are the guidelines according to the Vitamin D Council:

Infants: 1,000 IU/day no more than 2,000IU

Children: 1,000 IU/day per 25lbs of body weight no more than 2,000

Adults: 5,000 IU/day upper limit 10,000 IU

You will hear me talk about this vitamin a lot. Make sure you child has a blood test to see if they are deficient. The results may surprise you. It is simply that important for developing bones, muscles, and the brain. It is also helpful in preventing cancer, autoimmune diseases, and hypothyroid. Studies linking Vitamin D and Hypothyroidism (underperforming thyroid) to migraines or headaches: (33) (34)(35)

You may be surprised to learn that **magnesium** deficiency has been linked to headaches, as well. According to the United States Department of Agriculture (USDA), nearly half of the people suffering from migraine headaches show to have a low amount of ionized magnesium in their blood. (36)

In my practice, I have found that the blood test does not always show a deficiency, and we may supplement anyway, and we are getting results. I do believe that you should have your labs drawn, along with calcium and metabolic panels. How much should you be taking? According to the National Institute of Health here are their guidelines for daily supplementation:

Infants to age 3: 40-80mg

4-6 years old: 120mg

7-10 years old: 170 mg

Adolescent to Adult Males: 270-400mg

Adolescent to Adult Females: 280-300

Pregnant Women: 320 mg

Breastfeeding Women: 340-355 mg

In the office, I tend to recommend more. Depending what is going on with the child, I may recommend 500-1000mg per day, taken at night. I always give it at night, as it will help them sleep. Taking too much magnesium can cause loose stools or diarrhea, so that is something to watch out for. If it happens, cut back on your dosage.

Not many people have heard the term **adrenal fatigue**, or if they have and talk to their pediatrician or endocrinologist about it, it is very easily dismissed or they say there is no such thing. Well, I am here to tell you there is such a thing and it has a connection to thyroid, Vitamin D, magnesium deficiencies, and headaches.

So, what exactly are adrenal glands and how do they contribute to headaches? The adrenal glands sit on top of your kidneys and are responsible for producing cortisol and sex hormones. Cortisol has been called the "stress hormone," and is responsible for regulating the body during stages of increased stress in life. There is a normal pattern that cortisol follows. It is the lowest at night, which is what makes you tired, and highest in the morning, which is what wakes you up.

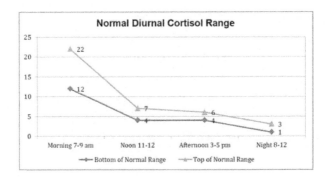

Due to our lifestyle, we always seem to be in a high state of stress. What that means is our cortisol is always high and does not come down as it should. There are some who have been so stressed for so long that their body can no longer produce cortisol due to exhaustion and stress put on the adrenal. When this happens, your children can't fall asleep or stay asleep, and they may experience headaches, weight gain, persistent illness, intestinal problems, and either irritable bowel syndrome or constipation. Many have light sensitivity, difficulty concentrating, lack of energy, the desire to sleep all day, mood swings, difficulty falling asleep at night despite exhaustion, and cravings. This sounds a lot like being in sympathetic mode, doesn't it?

Many of you may be saying to yourselves, "This all sounds like me." You are probably right. I myself have suffered with this and gone from doctor to doctor, hearing them tell me that nothing is wrong and that my labs are normal. I was getting adjusted on a regular basis so I felt like my systems were in a good place, but it wasn't until a fellow chiropractor educated me on adrenal fatigue that I was able to resolve it. I had a feeling it was adrenal related, but I didn't know how to fix the problem. I don't want anyone to have to experience the same runaround, which is why I am putting this in the book, for you to be more aware of it. I am seeing a higher number of children with adrenal fatigue than I should, meaning they are under an unhealthy amount of pressure and stress.

So how do you test for cortisol? The quickest way is through blood testing. You can do an AM and PM cortisol test, but it is not a complete test. The best way is through saliva and it is a test you do at home. Your child will spit into tubes throughout the day, and when completed, you send it off to a lab and they will plot it out and analyze it for you in a graph, as seen above. Correcting the adrenal does not happen overnight. It will take time. There are many products out there to help support the adrenals. In the office, I have seen the best results with Apex Energetics and Standard Process to get you started.

Many people benefit from (once again) a **gluten-free** diet, as it helps to keep the inflammation down. Others find a dairy-free and processed-sugar-free (natural sugars are okay), or Paleo diet helpful, as well. If your child does not feel better removing gluten or dairy, we may need to do a food sensitivity panel to see if there is something that your child is allergic to.

Let's recap on what labs you should be asking your pediatrician, functional medicine doctor, or chiropractor to be ordering:

- **Complete Metabolic Panel**

- **Lipids**

- **CBC**

- **Vitamins D and B's**

- **Magnesium**

- **Iron and ferritin**

- **AM and/or PM Cortisol**

- **Hemoglobin A1C**

- **For Thyroid: TSH, Total T3 and 4, Free T3 and 4, Thyroperoxidase TPO (for Hashimoto's)**

***Functional ranges of labs are listed in Chapter 10: Mood Swings.

Hashimoto's is an autoimmune disease of the thyroid. It is where the thyroid develops antibodies and will, in turn, attack itself. If left untreated, this can result in thyroid cancer, which is growing at an alarming rate. I have not seen it in a lot of children yet, but I am certainly seeing it a lot in young adults. (37)

The sooner your child is tested, the sooner you can know and make changes. Depending on who you talk to, most doctors will say there is "no cure" for Hashi's. By their typical practices and standards, they are right; there is no medicine to treat it, in other words. How you correct it is through diet and supplements, like L- Glutamine to repair the gut.

That means a very strict Gluten-Free diet, full of organics, and as GMO-free as possible. If you have ever heard the term "Leaky Gut," Hashimoto's and other autoimmune diseases are the consequences of our poor American diet.

Leaky Gut is what happens when proteins break through the intestinal barrier and get into our blood stream, usually due to an imbalanced bacteria or dysbiosis causing inflammation.

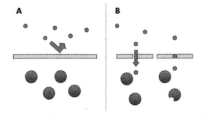

A: no disease. B: Intestinal permeability causing disease and autoimmunity (38).

The proteins are not supposed to leave our intestinal track, and the body produces antibodies to attack the foreign substances in the body, creating an immune response (autoimmunity). (38) The thyroid then comes into play by protecting the mucosal lining during stress, and can help to prevent ulcers (39). It is also where T4 (thyroxine) converts into active form T3 (triiodothyronine) in the gut and liver. Having poor bacteria in the gut can decrease the T3 and increase cortisol production from the adrenal glands.

Many people who are taking medication for their thyroid still are not feeling better, and the missing link is the gut connection. The diet must be cleaned up!! I would also incorporate probiotics along with some digestive enzymes to help with balancing out the gut.

Headaches can be one of the harder symptoms to pinpoint. They can come from nowhere, and can be so many different things or a combination of alignment and food allergies, or even something else. In the office, I always start with chiropractic alignments and go from there. That way I know that the body is balanced, and I can start looking at what else is going on biochemically in the body.

Quick Reference for Headaches

1. Just Water

2. Snacks and eating regular meals

3. Chiropractic care

4. Lab work

5. Supplements

6. Change in diet—Avoid trigger foods

CHAPTER 8

WHY DIDN'T MY PEDIATRICIAN TELL ME ABOUT CORRECTING POSTURE?

Posture is one of the single most important things to help keep your child healthy and happy into adulthood. I know we talked a little about it in the headache chapter, but here we are going to go more in depth. The sooner the problem is identified, the easier it is to correct, and that will carry into adulthood. Your body is designed to be balanced, which is why we have two arms, legs, eyes, nostrils, breasts, and ears on the body. Whereas at the midline of the body, we only have one heart, mouth, nose, stomach, liver, and bowel. Your body craves balance. What happens the body is out of balance?

Headaches, colds and flu, poor sleep, and later in adulthood can lead to knee and hip replacements from walking with more pressure on one side or the other, and of course neck and back pain (which affects over 31 million Americans at any given time) (40).

Everyone says that it's just "old age." Well, your right knee is the same age as your left knee, so old age isn't the problem; it's your body being out of alignment. You align your car on a regular basis so that it runs and functions at its best, and if you don't, what happens? Your tires will wear more on one side than the other. So why wouldn't you align your body? What are the biggest culprits of the decline in posture? Well, it all depends on who you talk to.

I say posture starts in the womb and whether or not mom had enough room for the baby to move and develop. Breech babies are becoming more and more common, and they shouldn't be.

More and more, women have sedentary jobs and sit at a computer the majority of the day. This cuts off the amount of room that baby has to develop and creates tight muscles, which is what we call **intrauterine constraint**.

Intrauterine constraint can lead to many developmental factors, including not enough room for the fetus to develop and flourish. Rotation of the hips and its muscles can lead to a baby not being in the proper position.

VARIATION IN FETAL PRESENTATION

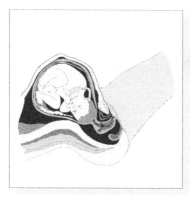
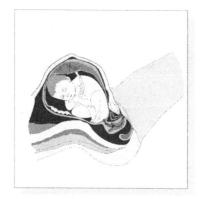

Cephalic presentation   Breech presentation

If you look at the picture above, you can see how the baby positioned properly has much more room, unlike the breech baby whose legs and arms are crammed together. The amount of pressure put on the baby's head in the breech position can cause the skull to be deformed (plagiocephaly), torticollis (head tilt), and lip- and tongue-tie.   It can also cause children to develop scoliosis. I have been seeing a big trend of children and young adults who have scoliosis, and I believe fetal positioning is partly to blame, along with a lack of nutrients.

There are many things you can do to help prevent having intrauterine constraint. Stretching and walking are wonderful. You should be walking 30-60 minutes per day. Yoga. Acupuncture. Massage and chiropractic care.

Try to find someone who is trained in the Webster Technique. According to the International Chiropractic Pediatric Association (ICPA), *The Webster technique is a specific chiropractic analysis and diversified adjustment. The goal of the adjustment is to reduce the effects of sacral subluxation/ SI joint dysfunction. In so doing neuro-biomechanical function in the pelvis is improved.*

You can find a provider at http://icpa4kids.org/Find-a-Chiropractor/ Also, make sure you are up on prenatal vitamins and supplements like Vitamin D and Omega-3 to help the baby's brain, bone, and muscle development.

Due to the increase in the number of moms with intrauterine constraint, I see so many children with **torticollis.** This is where the baby's head may be rotated and tilted to one side. Many children have a hard time breastfeeding, sleeping, and may be fussy. The standard care from a pediatrician is to do nothing right away, then start a program of physical therapy once they turn 1 year old, with the therapy lasting 6 months to a year, and the issue still not being resolved.

If your child has torticollis, you do not want to wait! Starting chiropractic care as soon as possible can help with cutting the therapy time in half. In my office, we usually see a complete resolution of torticollis within 6-8 weeks, other methods can take upwards of a year or longer. This is because I can get to the root of the problem with the spine being out of alignment, in addition to working and strengthening the muscles.

Please, get your child to a pediatric chiropractor; it will save you time and money!

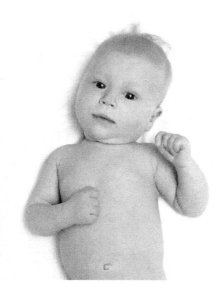

After birth, the best way help with an infant's posture is a lot of tummy time. This will help to build strong neck and core muscles for the future, help with hand-eye coordination, and help the developing brain to master motor skills.

A study in 2004 found children with more

experienced prone sleeping, displayed advanced motor skills, compared to those children that had less time on their bellies. The babies who were experienced with prone sleeping were able to lift their head and turn, versus those babies who lacked tummy time. (41)

In another study, they found prone positioning helped with babies rolling and sitting up sooner, whereas there was a lag in these motor skills for those babies that were laying on their backs. (42) At first your baby will not be happy, and you may only be able to do 1-2 minutes of laying on their belly. They will become frustrated in the beginning, but as the neck and core muscles begin to develop, your baby will be happy to stay on their stomach for a longer stretch of time.

Make tummy time fun by getting a play mat with things for them to look at. Mirrors are great, too. If you have other children in the house, have them talk to you baby as they are lying on their tummies, too. The more tummy time, the more a baby wants to crawl.

Crawling is one of the best ways for a child's body to develop both physically and mentally. Crawling helps to develop coordination, eyesight, tactile and spatial skills, and will strengthen the arms, shoulders, and spine. Do not allow your child to skip this phase in life! I have many parents who brag about how their children went straight to walking, and we are seeing that many of these children have a delay in motor skills, poor coordination, and also have a history of ADD/ADHD. Crawling is so important for the hand eye coordination as well and creating cross crawl patterns for the brain to connect the right and left hemispheres and be balanced.

You do not want your child to be dominate in one hemisphere over the other. There should be a nice balance. Crawling is not a guarantee that your baby will not have some sort of delay, but anything you can do to help prevent early on can only help in adulthood.

What are some things you can do to encourage crawling? While the baby is on their back, you can take their right hand and their left foot and bring them together, this is called **Cross Crawl.**

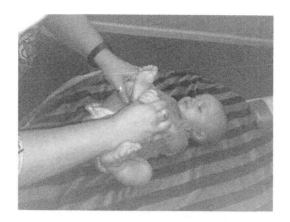

This is helping to stimulate the brain as a whole and to stimulate the nervous system. This is why walking and swimming are so important, as these activities require the use of both arms and legs in a crossing pattern, and I recommend these activities to many of my children who skipped the crawling phase. You should do these at least 3 times per day at 15 reps on each side.

Another way to encourage crawling is while your child is on their belly, put your hand behind their feet, and encourage them to push off. Start with them doing both feet at once, then do one foot at a time to push off.

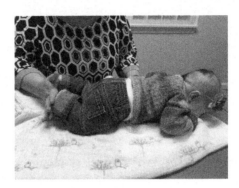

If you see there is a weakness on one side or the other, then spend more time on that foot. If you do not see an improvement, then seek out a pediatric chiropractor to have them evaluated for a pelvic or sacral misalignment.

Another way to help posture in the early years is by **wearing your baby** the proper way. I interviewed Heather Felker, CBE, Certified Baby Wearing Educator and owner of Sling with Me, a boutique for baby wearing and cloth diapering in Milford, DE, on what is the best way to wear a baby, and the reasoning why wearing a baby facing toward you versus away from you.

"When a baby is born, they enter the 4th trimester, and a baby expects constant contact. Baby wearing is not a benefit; it is actually the normal for the baby's needs. Carrying a baby in optimal position will help for spine (supports the kyphosis, vertebrae, and musculature to develop the normal "S" on the spine) and hip development. The position is called the **Newborn Tuck or Spread Squat.** <u>Knees above the bottom at a 45-degree angle</u>, it is the same angle as the harness used for hip dysplasia."

Heather also points out reasons why facing outward is not the most optimal:

1. Physiology of head and trunk development. They do not have the strength to face outward.

2. Kyphotic spine not developed and their back is towards a curvy parent.

3. As the child becomes older, now 20 pounds, the center of gravity is shifted on the parents. Parents' posture becomes an issue.

4. Socially lost contact of the face with parents. Babies have no basis of reaction to scenarios around them. They cannot see how parents react to a person coming

to the door. Are they a friend and happy, or should they be more cautious and serious?

5. Legs are not kept on Spread Squat.

6. Overstimulation. Babies can experience this in different ways. Some you will not be able to put own for a nap, they are up crying, or just can't keep their eyes off of things in the real world. Or, they can be so sleepy that their brain shuts down because of all the overstimulation.

7. Germs. Facing outward, your baby is exposed to more germs. Inward, they have a parents bubble and are not as exposed.

8. Kangaroo Care, the benefit of skin-to-skin, encourages breastfeeding, helps to

regulate body temperature.

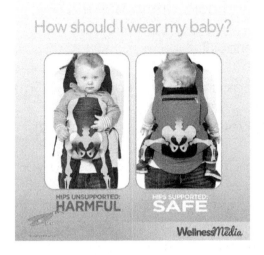

Mrs. Felker also went on to say, "Baby wearing can help to improve torticollis and plagiocephaly because parents can encourage babies to turn their heads, as opposed to car seats, where the baby is static." She helps to teach parents about posture and how to effectively turn the baby's head.

You can see there is an importance of spine and hip development in the early years, and wearing your baby improperly can hinder development later in life.

As your child is growing, what are some things you should watch out for? We are now in the technology world. Texting, iPads, video games, excessive sitting in school (student syndrome), and general lack of movement.

I can feel my posture changing as I am writing this book! It is a continual battle with keeping a strong core and good posture in today's society. Just take a look at your child. Have them take their shirt off and stand behind them.

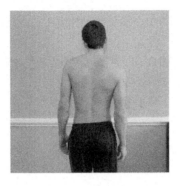

High Left Shoulder. Heat tilt to the Left. High Right Ear. High Right Hip.

What do you see? A high shoulder? A tilted head? Are their ears even? Do you see rotation in their body? Are their hips even, or is one higher than the other? From the side, is their head over their shoulders? Are they leaning forward?

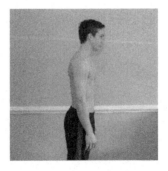

Head in front of shoulders. Forward lean.

242

Your child's posture is a window to the future!

Does your child look like this when sitting playing video games? See the rounding of the shoulders, and the head not over his shoulders? It looks like this child has a hunchback. This child more than likely, if he doesn't have them already, will be prone to headaches, may need glasses, will experience focusing problems, and will have chronic neck and shoulder pain. He probably isn't going to the bathroom on a regular basis, so he isn't sleeping well and is hard to get up in the morning.

With video games, not only does the child have

poor posture while playing, the games are over

stimulating and can cause stress (refer back to

the headache chapter for more on the

sympathetic nervous system).

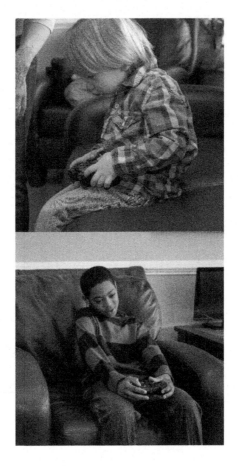

What about **Text Neck.** It's a real thing. When

you are looking at your phone or tablet, the more you look down, the more weight and pressure you put on your spine. How do you think you and your child are going to feel year after year of looking at texts?

On average, we are spending 2-4 hours per day looking down at our phones, and children are looking down longer because they are in school looking at books and schoolwork. Your head normal weighs the same as a bowling ball (10-12 pounds). Looking down at 15 degrees, your head now weighs as much as 2 bowling balls. At 60 degrees, your head can weigh as much as a toddler by adding an extra 50 pounds of pressure onto the body!(43)

Sadly, this is the state of our society, and there is no end in sight. Some of the symptoms of text neck are headaches (first and foremost), numbness and tingling in arms and hands, poor vision, and lack of focus just to name a few.

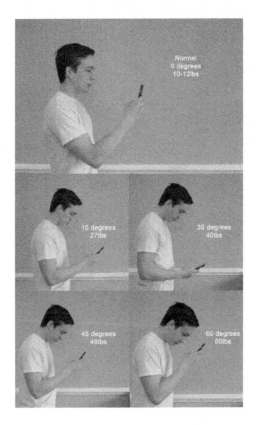

What can we do to help our children and

ourselves? Move! Get outside. Play with your kids, stimulate their brains. Engage their core muscles. Strong core muscles mean a strong back. If you see your child slouching when they are sitting at the table or playing video games, you need to correct them.

Limit the time they are allowed to play games or look at their tablet. If studying, make them get up at least every 20-30 minutes to stretch and take a break. Proper posture can be hard to encourage because, to a child, it feels uncomfortable. This is mainly because the core has weakened.

To strengthen muscles and improve posture when playing video games or sitting for extended times, have them sit on a **yoga ball**.

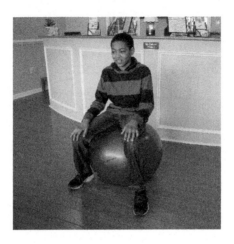

This can help with so many things. It helps to strengthen the core muscles, because if they have poor posture, they will fall off of the ball.

Sitting on a ball will help to stimulate the brain more, and cause them to have more focus. Just slight bouncing can release brain neurotransmitters more so than sitting in a chair. Studies show it can also help with better concentration at school, better behavior, and legible word productivity. (44)

One of my favorite exercises for children and adults is a **high plank**. Instead of using your forearms, you are up on your hands like you are going to do a push-up. This is a whole-body strengthening exercise. It works the core and back, as well as the arms and legs. The goal is to build up to a minute. Your child may only be able to do 10-20 seconds at first.

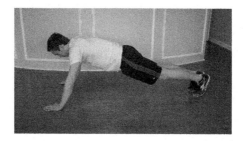

When that becomes easy, you can do

alternative planks and core. You can do low planks, use a ball, or a Bosu Ball.

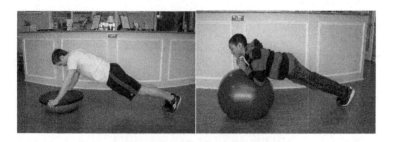

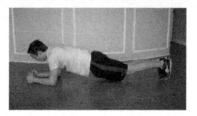

The Superman is another great exercise. You start out on your belly and raise arms and legs off the ground. You will want to build up to 1 minute If your child is not coordinated enough, then do this alone. If that is too hard, you can always do arms behind. Some children find it easier.

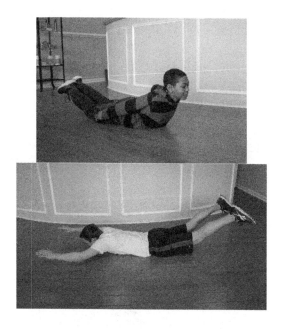

If your child has plenty of coordination and can follow directions, then you can add in the banana. You do this back and forth and make a game out of switching from superman to banana.

How to do the banana: lay on your back and raise both arms and legs off the ground at the same time. If doing the banana alone you will want to build up to 1 minute. If doing both Superman and Bananas together and switching back and forth, you will want to do this for 2 minutes.

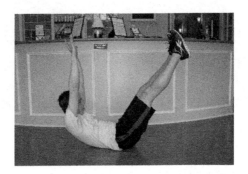

The next, and one of the harder exercises, is a back, core, and coordinating exercise. Parents will have to help initially because this exercise really challenges the child's balance. To begin, the child is on their hands and knees, and they will raise right arm and left leg straight out. Then, hold for 10 seconds. Then switch. This time, the

left arm is raised and the right leg is extended.
This will help to stretch the spine and its muscles,
while engaging the core muscles.

At first, this will likely be very difficult. You may
need to help support the arm and leg in the
beginning. You want to make sure there is
limited rotation of the hips. Kids will get frustrated
easily, but keep encouraging them. They will do
great!

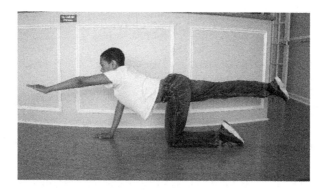

Earlier in the chapter we talked about cross crawl

for infants, now we will talk about how to do this for older children. Have them stand, and then bring the left hand up, and bend the right knee up so that they are only standing on their left foot. Their left hand will then touch their right knee as the knee is coming up, and the arm crosses the midline of the body. Then you will switch.

You will want to do 15-20 reps on each side, minimum three times per day. The Cross Crawl should not be rushed. The movements should be slow and deliberate. If you have a child with ADD/ ADHD, you may want to do this exercise more often. It can help to calm them down and focus, and may also help them to sleep better.

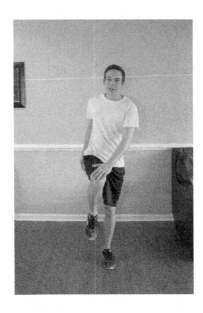

For some children, this will be hard at first. If they become too frustrated doing it while standing, then have them lay down. They can touch their right hand to their left foot, and then switch. Once they master the motions laying down, then have them start doing the exercise upright. Once upright becomes easy, then have them close their eyes.

You have to stretch your hamstrings and quads on a daily basis! We sit too much, and this will help! This will also help to keep the pelvis in alignment. I like having kids put their legs up on something like a box, table, stairs; anything to raise the leg off the ground. Then have them try to touch their toes. This stretch isolates the hamstrings and does not pull in the back too much.

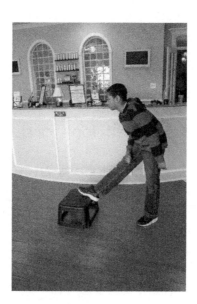

Stretching the quads you can do a few different ways. You can sit on your knees and lean backward, or you can stand on one leg while bending the other leg and grab the foot behind you with both hands.

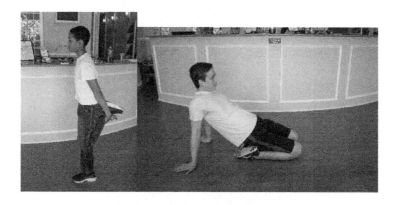

A great stretch to help with student syndrome and text neck is to so a doorway or wall stretch. These will help to stretch the pectoralis major and minor muscles that have become shortened while sitting. Depending on the age, you may have to pick either the wall or door. For older children, have them put both arms out to the side and lean forward. When doing this, have them look up to the celling.

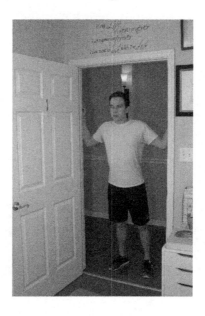

For smaller children, you may want to use the wall. With this method, they will do one arm at a time. Have them put their right arm on the wall and do a slight rotation until they feel the muscle stretch. The can move their arm up and down the wall at different angles to deepen the stretch.

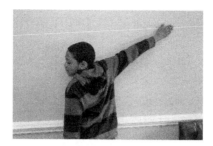

If you happen to have a yoga ball, you can also have your child lay over it backward with palms facing up and head back. This will also help to strengthen the core muscles while stretching pectoral and neck muscles.

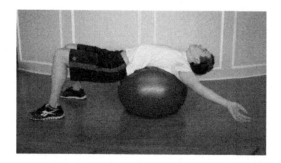

Once again, chiropractic adjustments will help

with posture, as well. I see babies from day one to get their tiny bodies in alignment and to start their life on the right path toward health and wellness. The sooner alignment is addressed, the better.

Even though children do not say they have neck and back pain, they still fall and sit all day, often don't eat the best, and are up late at night. This is creating the recipe for poor health, which may not show up until adulthood. I said it once, and I will say it again: <u>Posture is a window to the future</u>! Start early and take a **PROACTIVE** role in your child's health!

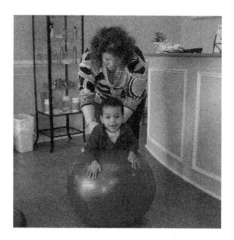

When adjusting children and adults, I always start with adjusting the pelvis and sacrum, since they are the foundation of your body. I explain to my patients the hips are just like a house foundation. If you build a house on an uneven foundation, the house falls apart over time little by little over time.

Proper alignment of the pelvis and hips keeps the knees, ankles, and feet strong and balanced.

This will in-turn help with allowing the head, neck, and shoulders to be in proper placements as well. Getting adjusted will help with reducing hip and knee replacements in the future, and maintain neck and shoulder placement. Regular adjustments will also help with keeping the lumbar and cervical spine stable and at a proper curvature. Here is what good posture looks like:

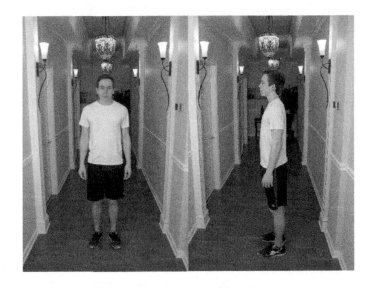

Ears over the shoulders, and shoulders in line with hips and knees. The better the posture, the healthier the child; fewer colds and flu, better focus and grades.

With all the talk about the structure of the body, you need to make sure you fuel and feed the body properly. Once again, gluten-free and dairy-free are the best scenarios since they are the most inflammatory to your body and its joints, but I know it is not for everybody.

If you do not wish to do either, then you need to watch for refined sugars in candy, breads, and cereals. Try to eat as much whole food as possible like fresh fruits and vegetables, and protein like fish and chicken.

Please eat organic as much as possible to limit

the amount of pesticides in plants, and hormones and antibiotics in animals.

As far as supplementing, we have talked about this so much in earlier chapters. The bare minimum is a good multi-vitamin. Omega-3's to support the organs, muscles, and ligaments. Vitamin D for overall body health. A good probiotic with at least 7-10 strains of good bacteria will help with your immunity, keep you and your child regular, and keep you from getting sick.

Quick Reference for Posture

1. Limit time sitting

2. Take breaks to stretch

3. Stretch and strengthen

4. Diet and supplements

5. Chiropractic adjustments

CHAPTER 9

WHY DIDN'T MY PEDITRICIAN TELL ME ABOUT HOW TO HELP MY CHILD WITH ADD/ADHD?

So many child these days are so quickly being diagnosed with ADD (Attention Deficit Disorder) or ADHD (Attention Deficit Hyperactivity Disorder) and no one looks into other factors, such as diet, sleep, and family lifestyle. Let's just medicate, and everything will be better, and you will be so happy your child is not getting in trouble anymore! ADD/ADHD, according to the Center for Disease Control, is one of the most common neurobehavioral problems in adolescent children.

Many doctors are ready to put children on medication so that they can focus better. I have some classrooms where 80-90% of the class is on some type medication for lack of focus. So who is benefiting from the medication, the children or the overstressed teacher who doesn't have all the resources to discipline in an overcrowded classroom? Should we be giving all this medication to a developing brain? I will be going through some alternatives to help your child with ADD/ ADHD.

ADD/ADHD can be described as an age-appropriate inattention. A child may or may not have impulsiveness or over-activity with their behavior. What are some of the signs your child may have ADD/ADHD?

- Not Focusing on the task at hand

- Fidgeting, constant moving around, restlessness

- Gets bored easily

- Thinking of a million things, mind racing

- Talking in class, or out of turn

- Not listening

- Forgetfulness

- Disorganized

- Procrastinating

- Loses things, especially schoolwork

This is not a complete list, but you get an idea. Why is there so much more ADD/ADHD today than ever before? Some would like to say we have better diagnostic tools to diagnose children. Some would say it's the foods we eat, the dyes, gluten, and the genetically modified (GMO) foods. Some would like to argue it's the TV and video games, and that kids just don't play outside like they once did.

So what's the answer? All of the above, plus more. How a child behaves begins before your child is born. It begins with their mom's and dad's diets. Were they healthy at the time of conception? Were they eating well, taking probiotics, and exercising? That all has to do with the chemistry and makeup of your child. Did you take Tylenol or acetaminophen during your pregnancy? If so, you have an increased chance of having a child with ADHD (45).

Vaccinations are also a hot topic to discuss. Overall, there have been no links to ADD/ADHD and vaccines. There is an online survey comparing vaccinated children to non-vaccinated children (there are no formal studies comparing the 2 groups), and ADD was at only 1-2% of children who were not vaccinated. (46) In an interesting research article that you should be aware of, looking at toxins such as lead, heavy metals (including thimerosal and Aluminum), and ethanol, played a part in developmental disorders such as autism and ADHD.

"Our studies also provide evidence that ethanol, heavy metals, and the vaccine preservative

thimerosal potently interfere with MS activation [dopamine-stimulated methionine synthase] and impair folate-dependent methylation.

Since each of these agents has been linked to developmental disorders, our findings suggest that impaired methylation, particularly impaired DNA methylation in response to growth factors, may be an important molecular mechanism leading to developmental disorders." (47) While further studies need to be conducted, it could be a factor in why we have seen an increase in Autism and ADD/ADHD (possibly due to the increase in the number vaccines our children are given since the 1980's.—See Wellness Chapter)

A recent case study found a link between Aluminum and Alzheimer's disease. (48) This is important to mention because aluminum is found in so many things, including drinks (pouches and cans), processed foods, foil, antacids, deodorants, and vaccines (including, but not limited to, Hepatitis A and B, Hib (Haemophilus influenzae type b), DTaP (diphtheria, tetanus, and pertussis), pneumococcal vaccine, and Gardasil (HPV)).

For a complete list of vaccines that contain aluminum and all their ingredients, please visit the Center for Disease Control and Prevention website www.cdc.gov/vaccines/vac-gen/additives.htm. Once aluminum is in the body, it is difficult to be removed. Aluminum is dangerous to the central nervous system and can cause brain inflammation and damage to the tissues, causing oxidative stress on the brain.

Over time, this leads to degeneration and is leading to Alzheimer's disease. Aluminum also targets the same part of the brain and nervous system for ADD/ ADHD, dementia, Parkinson's, and Autism.

When looking at the Material Safety Data Sheet of Aluminum, you will see some of the toxicity is the same as the neurological diseases and disorders. They include but not limited to:

- Memory problems

- Delay in motor skills

- Depression

- Speech impairment

- Seizures

- Muscle weakness

- Chronic fatigue

Aluminum tends to block glutathione, which is one of the best and important cellular detoxifiers and helps to lessen oxidative stress. Mercury comes into our bodies from the flu shot, as well in some fish, and glutathione is needed to help rid our bodies of the known neurotoxin.

Guess what else depletes glutathione? Tylenol or

acetaminophen, some of the most common analgesics given during pregnancy and childhood. It is routinely given after vaccinations and circumcision. By combining both vaccinations and acetaminophen, both which lead to glutathione depletion, there is an increase not only with ADHD and Asthma but also with Autism spectrum disorder (ASD). (49)(50) So it is best to try and limit your intake during pregnancy, and also limit giving it to your children, if possible.

The foods your child eats can also contribute to ADD/ADHD. While many look at dyes and sugars, yes these can cause focus issues,(51) I like to look at gluten first. **Gluten** and grains are very inflammatory for the whole body. Gluten is that "gluey" substance (protein) that is found in the wheat grain. It can be especially inflammatory more on the brain to some people. If the gut is healed, then the inflammation of the brain and body will go down.

For some children, we do lab testing for gluten sensitivity or those who have **Celiac's disease** (the disease is a reaction to gluten causing the mucosal lining in the intestines to be damaged). Celiac's is an autoimmune disorder where the body begins to attack itself. While once thought not to be very common in the United States, the numbers could be as high as 1 in 33 people. (52)

Your children need to be tested to find out for sure. The remedy is to completely remove gluten from the child's diet. There is a strong link to gluten and ADHD, and studies show a gluten-free diet is beneficial for children with ADD/ADHD. (53)

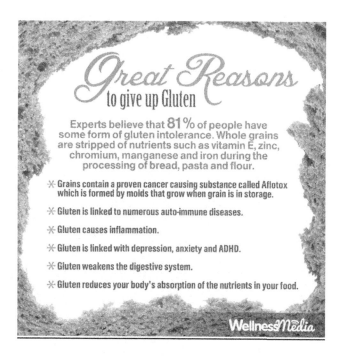

I also like to do food sensitivity panels on children with ADD/ADHD. I have found a lot of children are allergic/sensitive to other foods (besides gluten), causing inflammation of the brain. I use the Professional Co-op or Alletess to do the lab tests, and the test is out-of-pocket, as insurance usually does not pay for the food sensitivity test.

I like to test for IgG or Immunoglobulin G antibodies, of foods. If there are a lot of foods that come up High on the IgG test, I take out the ones that have the higher numbers first. It is always hard to say whether you are reacting to the food or are you having a reaction to a parasite or bacteria in the food, because an IgG response is fighting off bacteria and/or virus.

Either way, you need to remove it from the diet for at least 6-8 weeks, and then you can try to introduce the food again and see how the body reacts. If a sensitivity comes up with a fruit or vegetable, then try introducing a local, organic produce. If it is meat or cheese, buy grass fed, organic, non-hormone and non-antibiotic products. This can help you to be more in control of what you are feeding your children.

You can always grow your own foods, as well, if you like to and have the time. Maintaining good gut health also includes taking a good **probiotic.** I would like for your child to be on a nice blend of strains with no less than 7-10 strains of bacteria. We should have a high balance of the good bacteria to bad bacteria, at about a 10:1 ratio.

Good microflora of the intestines for a child with ADHD is important because the <u>serotonin</u> is produced in our gut. Serotonin is a neurotransmitter that is responsible for our mood and has been linked to depression. Describing the gut as our second brain is not far off. Serotonin is only found in the gut and not in the brain, so how your intestines feel determines how you will feel. When you have not gone to the bathroom for a few days, how do you feel? Bloated, irritable, cranky, and just not in a good mood in general. Increasing serotonin will help with improving brain function and mood.

In addition to probiotics and a better diet, you can also increase serotonin by being exposed to **bright light** and **exercise**. Please get your children outside and play! Running and jumping helps to stimulate the production of serotonin, and to improve your child's mood and brain chemistry. We sit too much and are indoors too much in today's society. (54)

Your child should be getting a minimum of 30 minutes of exercise per day. That can be running, playing tag, or going to the park. You want them to increase their heart rate. Jumping will help not only in increasing serotonin, but also drain their lymph nodes. The lymph nodes are important in maintaining a healthy immune system, as they filter foreign particles such as bacteria and viruses. Keeping the lymph drained properly will help keep your child's immune system boosted, so they are less sick.

Every morning, my daughter Madelyn and I put on her favorite songs, and we jump and sing and be silly. We have a small trampoline in the living room that she jumps on, and we take turns. I send her to school in a great and happy mood, plus her lymph is drained and her serotonin is boosted!

We cannot talk about serotonin without talking about **B vitamins**. B vitamins, especially B12 and Folate (B9), play an important role in serotonin production. They contribute to the production of SAM-e, or S-adenosylmethionine. This is a compound that helps to improve immune function, as well as produce serotonin. A simple blood test can be conducted to see where your child's levels are.

B12 levels should be at least 600 or above, and folate should be above 15. Depending on where the numbers are, I may do a B12 by itself, or I may suggest a B-complex supplement. We tend to have more folate since it is fortified in many of the foods we eat. Also, B12 is not found in plants, only in meats and dairy, which is why many vegetarians easily become B12 deficient.

When looking at lab work, should your child have a high folate and a low B12, you may want to investigate further. There is a gene mutation called Methylenetetrahydrofolate reductase, or MTHFR, and this helps to process amino acids for proteins, and requires folate to aide in the cycle. There are 2 possible mutations; C677T and A1298C, and there are a lot of scenarios that can occur. They could have one gene, both, or a set from each parent.

A simple blood test can determine if your child has the mutation or not. The gene has been linked to anxiety, depression, ADHD, headaches, bipolar, autism, miscarriages/infertility, and heart disease. Should your child happen to have this genetic mutation, they may benefit from a methylfolate instead of a folic acid due to the fact that, with the mutation, it is hard to break down folic acid. So, it may be worth it to have the test run to see genetically what is happening in your child's body.

What I have experienced in my office is many of my parents with children with ADD/ADHD say they cannot get their child to cut out sugar. They are addicted and a "sugarholic". Some parents say they are obsessed with candy, and will even have meltdowns if they do not get it.

These behaviors point to **yeast and candida.** Both yeast and candida (a yeast-like fungus) have to do with the microflora of the gut, and they live for sugar! Most commonly, they come from our American diet of high carbs with high gluten properties, and repeated antibiotics, causing yeast overgrowth. Once again, you can do a lab test to see if your child has either or both. Also, have your child stick out their tongue. Is there a white coating?? That is a sign of yeast or gut imbalance.

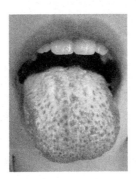

Getting rid of yeast and candida takes some time. You must remove sugar from the diet since that is what they thrive on. Cutting out carbs/grains and gluten; anything containing yeast. Adding coconut oil to your diet helps to naturally aid in yeast die off. I also encourage my patients to take a product called Yeastonil from Apex Energetics, which helps speed up the process. There may be some bloating, gas, itching, and skin may have some breakouts, but it is temporary. As both the yeast and candida die off, you will notice better behavior from your child.

In addition to yeast and candida, sugar cravings also have to do with dopamine. Dopamine plays a part in the reward system of the brain. Addictive drugs play a role in increasing the neurotransmitter in the beginning. The more you take, the more dopamine is produced, but its receptors become less receptive or responsive to the drug, in this case, sugar. Over time, the dopamine begins to diminish and then ADHD and overeating begins to happen (55). The following picture shows you images of different brains of people who are addicts (prolonged exposure to a substance over time). The normal MRI of the brain is dopamine, and as you can see, over exposure lessens the dopamine in the long run. If you were to test a child's dopamine levels, they would be low, and more than likely experiencing symptoms of ADD/ADHD.

Ritalin the most common drug prescribed for

children with attention issues helps to boost up dopamine. You have to change the diet first and foremost!! There is nothing fun about getting a child off sugar, and as you can see from the image, it is like getting someone off of cocaine. You will expect to have some outbursts and lashing out. You may have to do this slow and over time. I hear the words in my office all the time, "the medication worked initially, but it isn't any more." And the reason for that is they did not change anything in the diet, while their child had an initial increase in dopamine.

The body once again got used to the medication and the sugar, so the body began to non-reactive to the medication, and now our children are being prescribed stronger and stronger medications.

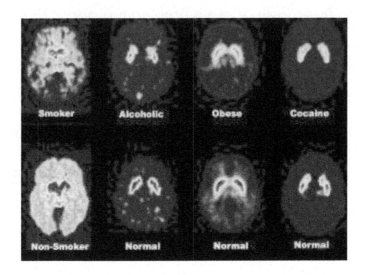

Image from Wikimedia Commons

There still seems to be a lot of speculation on whether or not sugar has anything to do with ADD/ ADHD, so further studies need to be done, and doing labs for yeast and candida can be conclusive. (55)

Fish oils and Omega-3's are talked about a lot when it comes to ADD/ ADHD. These are the good oils and fats that your body and brain need. As a nation, we are void of the good oils, and we tend to have a higher concentration of Omega 6's versus the 3's.

Adding omegas into the diet has been shown to help with inflammation of the body. Research on omegas and the benefits on helping children with ADD/ADHD have been mixed. Some have found them to be helpful while other studies have not.(56)

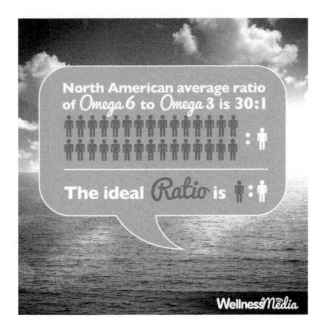

My experience with omegas has been positive, and we have seen great results in my office for children and adults alike. We use Nordic Natural's brand of omegas, as they are one of the best on the market and hold themselves to high standards. I usually recommend 1-3,000mg per day as a supplement, but your child can certainly eat cold water fish several times a week if they will. Not only are omegas great for the brain, but also for your heart, skin, and sight, and but they help to lower cholesterol, as well. There are so many benefits of omegas; we should all be supplementing.

It also has been noted that children with problems focusing are **zinc** and **magnesium** deficient as well. (57) Zinc plays a role in our immunity, and as well as aids in memory function. Zinc helps to activate over 100 enzymes in our body, including how our neurons communicate to one another.

It also plays a major role in the metabolism of

melatonin (aids in sleeping), which then regulates dopamine (the part of the brain that controls the reward and pleasure center as well as regulating movement and emotions). (58) Children with a lack of focus tend to have lower dopamine levels and have a hard time falling asleep or staying asleep.

It is important to note that the drugs used for ADD/ADHD all increase the production of dopamine. Parents who bring their children in to me usually do not want to give medications or are tired of how the meds make their children act, so zinc is another option.

By increasing zinc, you can increase melatonin

and dopamine at the same time. I recommend between 4-6mg for a child, and up to 12mg for a young adult or adult. If they are sick, you can double it when the immune system is down, but ONLY if they are not feeling well. I like my patients to take zinc at night to help them sleep. Our bodies do not take much zinc to run properly.

Magnesium's role in helping children with ADD/ADHD is that it helps to calm the nerves and muscles down. Many children are intense and experience tight muscles, they are not sleeping well, and have shifts in their blood glucose levels. Magnesium helps to regulate all of these things, and it is unfortunate that most doctors do not test for this mineral. It is involved in over 300 enzyme systems, so it is a major mineral needed for our bodies. Our children are becoming deficient due to a few factors. Sodas blocks magnesium from being absorbed. Also, high-sugar diets can hinder magnesium from staying in the body. Sugar, along with diuretics, cause the body to excrete magnesium in your urine, thus becoming deficient.

Processed foods and foods high in gluten, such as breads and pastas, are low in magnesium content. I usually recommend 250-500mg of magnesium for children, and around 1,000mg for young adults to and adults each day, depending on what is in their multivitamin. I also will want your child to take this at night with the zinc to help them sleep. The only downside to keeping an eye out for is too much magnesium can cause loose stools or diarrhea. If you child is experiencing this, simply halve the dose. Usually, it isn't a problem because the kids are so deficient, but it's just something I want you to be aware of.

Coenzyme Q10 (CoQ10) ubiquinone or ubiquinol, is also another supplement you may want to consider. It works well with magnesium and helps with providing energy to cells organs and muscles need. It is also considered an antioxidant.

Most of the time people associate heart health

with this supplement. While there is little research on CoQ10 and ADHD, I have found it to be beneficial in many of my patients; many parents say they notice a difference in behavior of their child.

We once again have to talk about **Vitamin D** because it's that important. Most of us have to supplement unless you are in a sunny state and can get your Vitamin D from the sun, with the best hours being between 12-2PM. For the rest of us, we will need to supplement, as little vitamin D comes from our foods.

Almost every cell in our body needs Vitamin D; it is essential to our heart, thyroid, and brain function. In a recent study, children with ADHD had lower Vitamin D levels as compared to normal school-aged children. I found the study disturbing because all of these children are deficient. The median number of the 1331 children in the ADHD group was 16, and for the other 1331 school-aged children, their D levels were 23. (59)

This goes to show you how deficient were are even as children, and that will carry on into adulthood. Studies have shown an increased risk of cancers, especially breast and colorectal, linked to low levels of Vitamin D, so it is imperative to maintain proper levels.(60)(61)

The level where the body functions at its best is between 60-80. And just like the other vitamins and minerals, a blood test is all that is needed to determine if your child is deficient. Here are the guidelines according to the Vitamin D Council:

- **Infants: 1,000 IU/day no more than 2,000IU**
- **Children: 1,000 IU/day per 25lbs of body weight no more than 2,000**
- **Adults: 5,000 IU/day upper limit 10,000 IU**

Chiropractic care should be part of your child's life (and yours) in helping them heal and recover with ADD/ ADHD, and studies (while small), are looking promising on helping children improve their focus.(62)(63)

By aligning and balancing the body, adjustments help to lower muscle tension and increase nerve and blood flow to the muscles, organs, tissues, and bones.

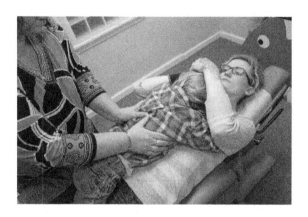

It also changes blood chemistry throughout the body and brain. Chemical, emotional, and physical stressors put strain on our bodies and can cause misalignments of the spine, causing us not to function at our best. Regular chiropractic adjustments will help your body to defend itself from the stressors that our bodies are always being exposed to. Some of the stressors includes:

- the American Diet (processed foods, GMO, high sugar)
- stress of school
- home life
- falls
- sports
- sick all the time: colds/flu/allergies
- medications
- vaccinations
- not getting enough sleep
- lack of proper nutrients: vitamin and mineral deficiencies
- dehydration; lack of water

All of these things put added stress on the body

and the stress can add up, but by getting alignments, your body can help to manage the stress more efficiently. Chiropractic adjustments are more beneficial when you add in changes to diet and adding in supplements to support the whole body. In addition to getting plenty of water and sleep, your body needs balance, fuel, and downtime to function properly.

One of my favorite exercises to help calm the brain (I show teachers how to do this in their classroom) is the **cross crawl**. The cross crawl stimulates the brain by utilizing both sides of the brain at the same time, creating a bridge between the two hemispheres. With so many of our children skipping crawling as a baby, missing this step and going straight to walking can hinder coordination, cause focus problems, and affect the nervous system's ability to communicate to the rest of the body, all of which can carry into adulthood.

Start by bringing your right arm up in the air with the left leg at the same time. Then bring your right hand to your left knee, crossing over the midline of the body. Then switch to do the left arm and right leg; you are making a lasting impression by strengthening the nervous system.

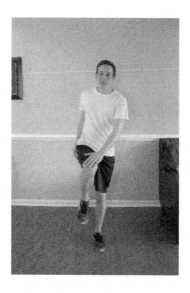

For many children in the beginning, this can be difficult because of lack of focus or coordination. Keep with it! It will get better, stronger, and easier with repetition. There will be times when your children will get frustrated with it. Take a break and come back to doing cross crawl later. You should plan on doing 15 reps on each side of the body 3 times a day. If at any time your child is not listening or won't sit still, have them stand up and do the cross crawl. I have teachers in class do this if the kids will not listen or they don't seem engaged. It changes their state of mind as well as strengthen it at the same time.

Other things you can do is stand on a **wobble board** or a **Bosu ball**. Both of these will help with balance and coordination. On the wobble board, stand with both feet even, and try to balance.

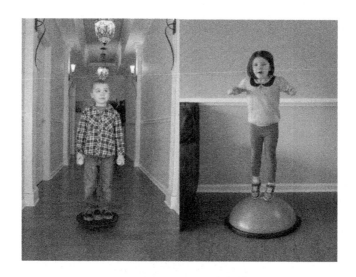

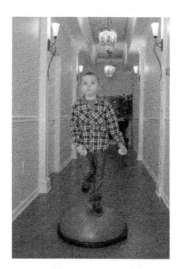

When that becomes easy, then stand with one foot in the middle of the board, and switch legs.

Both of these exercises help to strengthen the core muscles as well as balancing the brain. I also like to use a **Power Plate.** They are great for circulation, drain lymph, and help to stimulate the brain. Kids love standing on it and an easy way to get them to do some exercises.

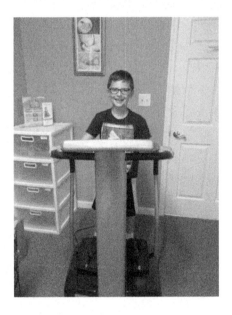

As you can see, there are lots of natural options

that can help your child with ADD/ADHD. You must give some of these changes time; it will not happen overnight. Be patient. Changes will happen!

Quick Reference for ADD/ADHD

1. Remove Gluten

2. Exercise

3. Bright lights

4. B and D vitamins

5. Omegas

6. Chiropractic

7. Remove sugar/yeast and candida

8. Zinc and Magnesium

9. Cross Crawl/wobble board

CHAPTER 10

WHY DIDN'T MY PEDIATRICIAN TELL ME

HOW TO CALM MOOD SWINGS?

Mood swings. There is nothing fun about them. How can our children go from being in such a great and happy mood to the point where their world has been turned upside down? We see outbursts in our young children, but more in our teenage girls. There are so many different things it could be, where do we start?

Usually when a parent brings in their child for behavioral issues, one of the first things we do is go through the diet. Almost always, we have to change several things. One of the biggest problems I encounter is children are severely dehydrated due to lack of water. Kids today drink a lot of sugary drinks including milk, juice, sodas, designer coffee, power drinks, as well as energy drinks that children have actually died from.

This is the easiest part of the diet to change, and you will see dramatic results just from changing this alone. If you can, you want to get to the point where there are no sugary drinks at all. I know this will not happen overnight, but do the best you can.

Water should be the primary drink of choice to

hydrate, and it helps with balancing the pH of the body. Sugar makes the body more acidic, which can lead to a cranky child. Once again the amount of water is **BODY WEIGHT/2**. A 100-pound child should be drinking 50 ounces of water per day. And if they are involved in sports, you should be increasing water intake by at least another 20 ounces.

When it comes to diet, more of a well-balanced approach is best. I know this is not always easy, especially if you have a picky eater in the house. I am all too familiar as with this. It is a struggle for us, as well. Try to get in as many fruits and vegetables as possible. They can have unlimited veggies, but try to keep the fruits that are high in sugar to a minimum. Berries such as blueberries, strawberries, and raspberries are low glycemic index fruits.

Apples, oranges, mangos, and bananas are higher in sugar so should be limited to a few times per week, as opposed to daily. Lean meats are preferred. Chicken, fish, turkey, whichever you prefer. Red meats should be limited to a few times per month. I prefer kids get their iron from green leafy vegetables such as spinach and kale.

Gluten found in pizza, pasta, bread, and crackers can cause an array of problems. The biggest problems I hear from children is that their stomach hurts and they have headaches. Many children with a gluten sensitivity have a hard time concentrating, too. While we are all sensitive to gluten to a point, I like to do a lab test to see exactly what is going on. You can do a single gluten sensitivity test or a full food panel to see what else your child could be sensitive to.

Like we talked about before with cutting out sugary drinks, you will want to **cut out processed sugar.** Sugar is very addictive and can act like an opiate (cocaine) on the brain. (64)(65) The red in the scan below is neurotransmitter dopamine. Dopamine's roll on the body includes: motor control, motivation, and the reward center of the brain. As you can see, both cocaine and sugar have the same amount of dopamine, which can cause children to have a delayed motor, not finding pleasure in anything(kids may say "this is stupid" or "this is boring"), and having cravings of sugar to help boost up the dopamine levels to feel good again.

Both cocaine and sugars initially help to increase dopamine in the short term, but then long term it takes more and more substances to get that "high" and eventually dopamine receptors will start to deplete so it will take more and more sugar to maintain dopamine. This can lead to overeating and obesity. Can you guess which medicine helps to boost dopamine?? Ritalin, the same prescribed for children with ADD/ADHD.

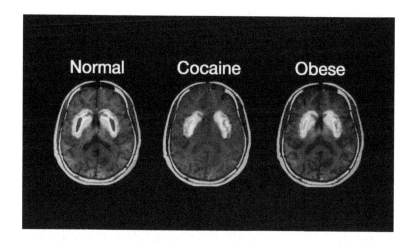

The higher your sugar intake, the more your body

wants it, which can lead to overeating due to all

of the cravings your body is signaling.

As your child starts to come off of sugar, just like

an addict, withdrawals can set in. There can be

some depression, outbursts, and anger, but they

will feel better in the long run, and these changes help to keep minds and bodies more alkalized. You can order test strips off the internet to test whether your child is alkaline or acidic.

You are striving for a Ph of 7.25. Within a short period of time, you will notice a difference in your child's behavior and see fewer mood swings.

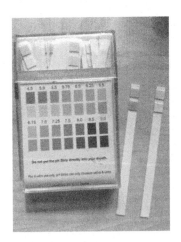

While changing some of the dietary changes, it is important to implement some **exercise**. Sweating is a great way to help flush the toxins out of the body, and it also increases your need for water. Encourage a brisk walk, jog, or even just getting outside and moving. Any kind of sport. Find something they will like and follow through on it. You can join a gym, go for hikes, and take the dog for a walk. Stay away from the television, because that will be a trigger for wanting to eat more sugary foods. Get the whole family involved. I know it isn't always the easiest, but do the best you can. Finding time for everyone to get together can be challenging. Set a few times per week when you can all meet. When you schedule a day and time, you are more likely to get it done!

You can also look into a small trampoline or a vibration plate for the house. Both of these can help with circulation on blood, help drain the lymph, and can help with detoxifying the liver. Just 10 minutes a day can greatly improve their immune system.

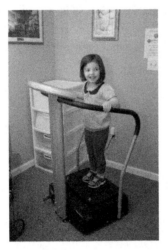 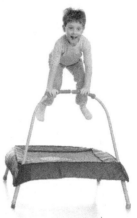

When talking about mood swings, we have to address how often your children **poop**. Moving your bowels helps to remove toxins from the body. When doing my exam, most children are not even pooping once a day, some not even once a week. No wonder they are cranky and miserable!

Getting the gut in balance will help with your children to become "regular." Many of the things you can do, we have already talked about. Increase water, more water-rich foods like fruits and vegetables, digestive enzymes, and exercise.

One of the best things you can also do for your child's belly is to give them **probiotics.** Just like all the other supplements there is no shortage of probiotics and yogurt isn't cutting it. We use

DaVinci brand in our office because of several reasons: It is vegetarian, and dairy-, GMO-, and gluten-free. It is also a capsule that comes apart, and can be given to children and adults alike. It contains 8 strands of different bacteria to help repopulate the gut with the good bacteria.

Poor gut flora is caused by a multitude of things, anywhere from high processed foods, anti-inflammatory drugs, medicines to stop acid reflux, antibiotics, as well as vaccines, can all decrease the good bacteria in our bodies. Introducing probiotics daily will help get things moving.

Also in dealing with sluggish bowels and mood

swings, doing some lab work can also narrow down and pinpoint a cause. Things I like to test for in the office is a **thyroid panel**, looking not only at thyroid stimulating hormone (TSH), but also looking at **T3** and **T4**, as well as antibodies of the thyroid.

More and more children are becoming hypothyroid (high TSH, sluggish and underperforming thyroid) and I am seeing children being put on medicine at an early age. The main reason is due to lack of nutrients and high processed foods. You should also have **Vitamin D** levels checked.

Checking for **yeast** and **candida** are options too.

Especially if they are <u>craving sugars</u> and are having an <u>acne</u> problem. Yeast and Candida is a sign of **Leaky Gut,** meaning small particles of bacteria, yeast, toxins, and foods pass through the stomach and intestine lining and go to the blood stream.

One of the major symptoms is mood swings, fatigue (because your body is not absorbing nutrients), and belly issues. A simple blood test for yeast and candida can be done. This is a great and reliable test to see if you have leaky gut. If they come back positive, then it is a good sign your child's gut needs to be overhauled because they are not to be found in the blood, only in the digestive tract.

<u>Getting rid of yeast and candida</u> take some time, but the biggest thing to do is to cut out sugars... They LOVE sugar. It fuels them and allows both yeast and candida to grow, so you have to cut off the food supply. No yeast products, gluten- and grain-free is best. 1-2 tablespoons of coconut oil will help, too.

If you can, have them eat it alone, but if not, put in a smoothie. Don't forget the probiotics, they are imperative to getting the good bacteria back into the gut. Also, there are several products out there for Apex Energetics called Repairvite (for leaky gut) and Yeastinol (for yeast and candida). Both are great products, and I use them in the office on a regular basis.

Also, have a **CBC**, a **complete metabolic Panel**, and a **Lipid panel**. I also like to check **magnesium**, even though it is not the most efficient way to check for the low mineral, it gives me an idea along with the symptoms the child is experiencing. Also I would check for **Gluten** like I had said before. This is a good place to start. You will want to look for these ranges in some of the labs. These are the best _Functional_ _Ranges_ where your body functions at its best:

- TSH: 1-2 mIU/L
- T3 total: 100-180ng/dL
- Free T3: 3.0-4.0pg/mL
- T4 Total: 6-12 µg/dL

- Free T4: 1.0-1.5 ng/dL

- Vitamin D 60-80 ng/mL not below 50

- Magnesium: 2.0-2.5 mg/dL

- Calcium: 9.6-10.1 mg/dL

- Glucose: 85-99 mg/dL

- Potassium 4.0-4.5 mmol/L

Supplements are an integral part of helping mood swings, and depending whether or not you did lab work, determines what you should supplement with. I like to start children on an **Omega-3's**, which are the long chain fatty acids containing docosahexaenoic acid (DHA) and eicosapentaenoic acid (EPA), which help with decreasing inflammation.

Our American diets are full of Omega-6's which is more inflammatory and causing aches, pains, and mood swings and thyroid problems. The benefits of taking fish oil are great for your organs, especially your heart and brain, and can help with reducing triglycerides.

You can get your Omegas from eating fish 2-3 times a week. Salmon and swordfish are great options. But you can also supplement, too. I like to use Nordic Natural Brand; it is one of the best out there. You will want to supplement with 1-3,000mg of Omegas per day. Many of my parents say they notice their children's hair getting stronger and not falling out as much. They also notice their children are focusing and sleeping better, as well.

Of course I'm going to talk about **Vitamin D** again. And with dealing with mood swings, your child must be taking a supplement or getting plenty of sun, depending on where you live. Lack of Vitamin D can cause tiredness, chronic pain, headaches, moodiness, poor bowels, and poor concentration. Sounds like many adults have the same problem.

Please have your physician check to see where yours and your child's levels are. For a young child, 1-2,000 IU daily should be plenty, while in a young adult, 3-4,000 IU will be enough. I prefer a liquid Vitamin D, and we use Xymogen in the office. We see great results, and parents say they see a difference within a few weeks.

Sodas are one of America's favorite drinks of all time, but it comes at a price. They contain phosphoric acid which depletes magnesium and can lead to an array of other deficiencies.

Magnesium is often a mineral that is overlooked, and much of America is low. It works in conjunction with Vitamin D, so it is only natural if your D is low, then you magnesium is, too. They have a symbiotic relationship. Magnesium helps with Vitamin D (66) and calcium absorption, but it is a fine balance because too much magnesium can inhibit Vitamin D absorption and vice versa.

A few common signs you are low in magnesium is craving nuts and chocolate. Low magnesium can cause some moodiness, but it can also cause painful and cramping menses/periods in teenage girls. There are several ways you can get magnesium: through foods such as leafy greens, almonds, cashews, or Brazil nuts. A little bit of dark chocolate can give you some magnesium, too.

You can also supplement, as well. I usually recommend Magnesium citrate and not a cal-mag combo. We get enough calcium in our diet because most foods are fortified with calcium. Toddlers you can supplement with around 100mg per day of magnesium. Young adults should receive 300-500mg per day. If you have a teenage girl with horrible periods, double up on the magnesium about 2-3 days before her period. This will help lessen the cramping.

A **mineral complex** is always a great choice since we are low in our minerals, between our foods (either being too processed, or our soil is not as nutrient rich as it once was), but also the lack of minerals in our multi-vitamins. Most multi-vitamins only contain around10 minerals. We use a liquid called Youngevity Cheri-mins in our office which has around 70 trace minerals your body needs on a daily basis.

B12 and Folate are essential in mood swings, as

they play an important role in producing serotonin, which is a neurotransmitter found in the gut and minimal in the brain, and is responsible for mood. This is another reason why we need to take care of the gut.

We talked about serotonin extensively in the ADD/AHHD chapter. A quick lab test can tell you more information if you child is low, and you can either supplement (methylcobalamin) or get B12 through meats and dairy, as they are not found in plants. Like I had said before, many vegetarians are lacking B12.

Our children are under so much more pressure than we were growing up. Children are under stress to perform at school (grades and standardized testing), to complete homework, to participate in sports or music lessons, plus work or babysitting- no wonder they are having mood swings!

The more stress, the higher cortisol levels are throughout the body and the increase in mood swings. You may notice your child gaining weight, having acne, and craving sweets and carbs. Also you may notice they are tired all day and may not be sleeping at night, or are having a hard time falling asleep. They could be having lots of colds, runny nose, and poor concentration. This could be **adrenal dysfunction** or **adrenal fatigue.** Our adrenal glands sit on top of our kidneys and play a role in so many different things that typically get overlooked. They produce several hormones.

- Cortisol--helps with metabolism and stress
- Aldosterone--helps control blood pressure
- Adrenaline--helps your body react to stress
- Sex hormones--small amount as compared to ovaries and testes

Cortisol should follow a pattern throughout the day. It should be highest in the morning, and slowly lowering at certain points of the day. Usually, around 11 in the morning and 3-4 in the afternoon, and it becomes the lowest around 10 in the evening when you are ready for bed. Low cortisol is what makes you tired, and when it increases through the night, it is what wakes you up in the morning.

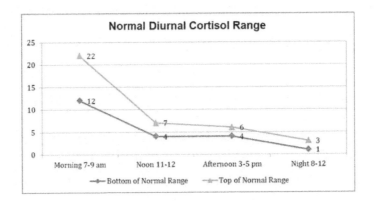

With adrenal dysfunction, we can tend to have high cortisol all throughout the day. When this happens, we have a slew of things that happen like I had talked about above. When the high cortisol becomes a chronic issue, there will become a point when the adrenal glands can no longer produce cortisol to keep up with demand, so it stops making cortisol, and this is termed **adrenal failure**. Having suffered with it myself, we want to control the cortisol before it gets to this point.

First we must find out if you child has an adrenal dysfunction to begin with. The best way to test is through saliva, and it is an all-day test. Your child will spit in tubes throughout the day at designated times. You will keep them in the refrigerator until you are ready to ship off. I like to use the company DiagnosTechs (www.diagnostechs.com).

Within a week, they will send you back a graph that looks similar to the picture above. It will have the normal range, and it will also plot where your child's numbers are. Typically at this age, the range should be normal but plenty are on the high side. If high, we then need to do relaxing techniques, some diet changes, and maybe an adrenal supplement to help lower the cortisol.

We have already talked about going gluten free and cutting out refined sugars, so some <u>relaxation techniques</u> that can even be done at school are easy.

Breathing is one of the easiest to do. Take deep breaths in through the nose and out the mouth, and drop the shoulders. Do this with your eyes closed. Just doing this alone will drop your cortisol. You can meditate, do yoga, or go for a walk. Do anything you find relaxing to help lower stress levels so the cortisol decreases.

When looking to low stress and overall feel better, regular **chiropractic adjustments** are a must. Many children with mood swings are not sleeping well, and just do not feel good in general. They just don't have the energy and vitality they should have. They have poor posture and a poor diet, so regular alignments of the body will help to restore and reset the body to balance.

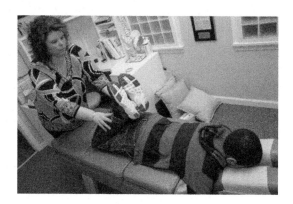

By aligning the body, biochemical changes take place to help bring the body to homeostasis. The body craves balance. An adjustment helps to stimulate the nervous system and wake it up. Your entire body is controlled by the nervous system, so proper and regular alignments will help to maintain the brain, spinal cord, and nerves.

With kids sitting so much these days, chiropractic is imperative to life. Our bodies are becoming dormant, so wake it up! Move! Regular adjustments will help with decreasing the inflammation in the body, help with balancing hormones, and help boost your child's white blood cell count, so children are less sick and maintaining a better immune system.

They will start to sleep better which will help to calm the brain down so they can actually get a fresh start in the mornings. A child dealing with mood swings will find that they feel better after an adjustment. A happier child means happier parents.

As you can see, it isn't just one thing that helps mood swings, it's a combination of many different pieces. You will have to find what works best for you and your child. The bottom line is clean up their diet, increase water intake, get adjusted, and exercise regularly. These will help with the mood swings.

Quick Reference for Mood Swings

1. Water

2. Cut out Processed Sugars

3. Exercise

4. Lab work

5. Vitamin D

6. Omega-3's

7. Thyroid and Adrenal Glands

8. Breathing

9. Chiropractic Care

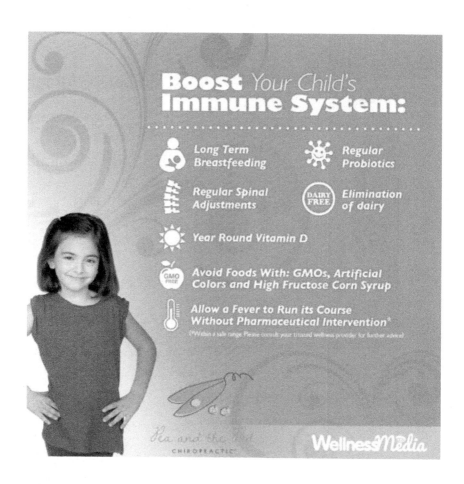

ABOUT THE AUTHOR

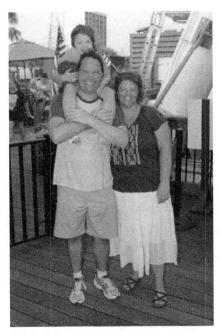

Dr. Brenda Fairchild is not your average chiropractor. She has a unique understanding, as well as personal experience that she infuses into every aspect of your journey while working with her.

She is the founder and practitioner of Pea and the Pod Chiropractic. After working in medicine for 12 years, Dr. Brenda found her calling in Chiropractic care where there is a more holistic approach. Upon completing school, she became pregnant with Madelyn Jaymes. Chiropractic care helped to heal her lower back pain and helped get Maddy into a better position so that she had the most room to develop her brain and spine. Dr. Brenda then became specialized in women's health, pregnancy, fertility, and pediatric chiropractic care.

She is one of the few chiropractors in the state of Delaware who is Webster Certified. She is Board Certified in Pediatric and Pregnancy Chiropractic Care through the International Chiropractic Pediatric Association and Academy of Family Practice.

Dr. Brenda loves spending time with her husband Joseph and daughter Madelyn. They love to travel and go to the "big city" as Maddy calls it for adventures. Also in the family are three miniature dachshunds: Hunter, Mousse, and Sparky, who love to take Maddy on walks.

Education:

- Post Doctorate, Board Certified in Pediatric Chiropractic and Pregnancy Care (CACCP)

- Parker University
  - Doctor of Chiropractic (DC)
  - Bachelor of Science Anatomy (BS)
  - Bachelor of Science Health and Wellness (BS)

- University of Nevada Las Vegas
  - Bachelor of Arts Sociology (BA)
  - Radiology Technologist Certificate (ARRT)(R)(M)

- International Chiropractic Pediatrics Association/Academy of Family Practice
  - Webster Technique Certification

- Certified Doula from Doulas of North America (DONA International)

- Certificate in Spinning Babies Workshop for pregnancy and breech education

Bibliography

1. Michaëlsson, K,. Wolk, A. 2014 Milk intake and risk of mortality and fractures in women and men: cohort studies. *BMJ* 349:g6015

2. Center for Disease Control and Prevention. 2015. Antibiotic Resistance Questions & Answers. www.cdc.gov/getsmart/antibiotic-use/antibiotic-resistance-faqs.html

3. Kent, Christopher. Models of Vertebral Subluxation: A Review. Journal of Vertebral Subluxation Research. August 1996, Vol 1:1. Pg 4-5

4. Pero R. Medical Researcher Excited By CBSRF Project Results. The Chiropractic Journal. 1989; 32.

5. Selano JL et al. The Effects of Specific Upper Cervical Adjustments on the CD4 Counts of HIV Positive Patients. The Chiro Research Journal. 1994; 3(1).

6. Vitamin D Council. 2015. https://www.vitamindcouncil.org/further-topics/vitamin-d-during-pregnancy-and-breastfeeding/#

7. National Institutes of Health (NIH). 2015. http://ods.od.nih.gov/factsheets/VitaminC-HealthProfessional/

8. National Vaccine Information Center. 2015. http://www.nvic.org/NVIC-Vaccine-News/August-2014/Back-to-School-Vaccines--Know-the-Risks-and-Failur.aspx

9. Kidd, Parris. 2003.Th1/Th2 Balance: The Hypothesis, its Limitations, and Implications for Health and Disease. Alternative Medicine Review ,Volume 8, Number 3. Pg. 223-246

10. Sult, T. Th1/Th2 Balance: A Natural Therapeutic Approach to Th2 Polarization in Allergy. Applied Nutritional Science Reports. http://www.afmcp-sa.com/ansr/ansr_index.html

11. Wiberg JM, Nordsteen J, Nilsson N. The short-term effect of spinal manipulation in the treatment of infantile colic: a randomized controlled clinical trial with a blinded observer. J Manipulative Physiol Ther. 1999 Oct;22(8):517-22.

12. Miller JE, Newell D, Bolton JE. Efficacy of chiropractic manual therapy on infant colic: a pragmatic single-blind, randomized controlled trial. J Manipulative Physiol Ther. 2012 Oct;35(8):600-7. doi: 10.1016/j.jmpt.2012.09.010.

13. Alcantara J, Alcantara JD, Alcantara J. The chiropractic care of infants with colic: a systematic review of the literature. Explore (NY). 2011 May-Jun;7(3):168-74. doi: 10.1016/j.explore.2011.02.00

14. Wagner CL, Hulsey TC, Fanning D, Ebeling M, Hollis BW. High-dose vitamin D3 supplementation in a cohort of breastfeeding mothers and their infants: a 6-month follow-up pilot study. Breastfeed Med. 2006 Summer;1(2):59-70

15. Wu,H, Wu, E. The role of gut microbiota in immune homeostasis and autoimmunity. Gut Microbes. 2012 Jan 1; 3(1):4-14

16. Kosiewicz, M, Zirnheld,A, Alard, P. Gut Microbiota, Immunity, and disease. A Complex Relationship. Frontiers in Microbiology. Publishes online 2011 Sept 5. http://www.ncbi.nlm.nih.gov/pmc/articles/PMC3166766/

17. Joneja, J. Carmona-Silva, C. Outcome of a Histamine-restricted Diet Based on Chart Audit. Journal of Nutritional & Environmental Medicine (2001) 11, 249–262

18. The National Association for Child Development. 2015. http://nacd.org/health/protocol.php

19. Schroeder, HA. Losses of vitamins and trace minerals resulting from processing and preservation of foods. The American Journal of Clinical Nutrition 24: MAY 1971, pp. 562-573

20. Langmead L, Feakins RM. Randomized, double-blind, placebo-controlled trial of oral aloe vera gel for active ulcerative

colitis. Aliment Pharmacology and Therapeutics. 2004 Apr 1;19(7):739-47.

21. Hendley, J. Otitis Media. New England Journal Medicine October 10, 2002. 347:1169-1174

22. Fallon, JM. The role of the chiropractic adjustment in the care and treatment of 332 children with otitis media. Journal of Clinical Chiropractic Pediatrics 1997;2(2):167-183

23. Froehle RM. Ear infection: a retrospective study examining improvements from chiropractic care and analyzing for influencing factors. J Manipulative Physiol Ther 1996;19:169-77.

24. Takeda, Y. Arai, S. Relationship Between Vertebral Deformities And Allergic Diseases. The Internet Journal of Orthopedic Surgery, Volume 2, Number 1. https://ispub.com/IJOS/2/1/8061

25. Bronfort G, Evans RL, Kubic P, Filkin P. Chronic pediatric asthma and chiropractic spinal manipulation: a prospective clinical series and randomized clinical pilot study. J Manipulative Physiol Ther. 2001 Jul-Aug;24(6):369-77.

26. Graham, R. Pistolese, R. An Impairment Rating Analysis of Asthmatic Children Under Chiropractic Care. Journal of Vertebral Subluxation Research.Volume 1. Number 4,Pg 1-8.

27. Center for Disease Control and Prevention. 2015. Antibiotic / Antimicrobial Resistance. http://www.cdc.gov/drugresistance/threat -report-2013/

28. Hodge, L. Salome, C. Peat, J. Haby, M. Xuan, W. Woolcock, A. Consumption of oily fish and childhood asthma risk. Medical Journal of Australia. 1996; 164 (3).

29. Kabbouche, M. Gilman, D. Management of Migraine in Adolescents. Neuropsychiatric Disease and Treatment. 2008 June; 4(3): 535-548.

30. Peroutka, SJ. Migraine: a chronic sympathetic nervous disorder. Headache. 2004 Jan;44(1):53-64.

31. McCrory, D. Penzien, D. Hasselblad, V. Gray, R. Behavioral and Physical Treatments for Tension-type and Cervicogenic Headache. Duke University Evidence-based Practice Center Center for Clinical Health Policy Research. The Foundation for Chiropractic Education and Research. http://www.chiro.org/LINKS/FULL/Behavior al_and_Physical_Treatments_for_Headach e.html

32. Tuchin, P. Pollard, H. Bonello, R. A randomized controlled trial of chiropractic spinal manipulative therapy for migraine. Journal of Manipulative and Physiological

Therapeutics. February 2000Volume 23, Issue 2, Pages 91–95.

33. Celikbilek, A. Gocmen, AY. Zarasiz, G. Tanik, N. Borecki, E. Delibas. Serum levels of vitamin D, vitamin D-binding protein and vitamin D receptor in migraine patients from central Anatolia region. International Journal of Clinical Practice. Volume 68, Issue 10, pg. 1272–1277, October 2014.

34. Moreau, TH. Manceau, E. Giroud-Baleydier, F. Dumas, R. Giroud, M. Headache in hypothyroidism. Prevalence and outcome under thyroid hormone therapy. Cephalalgia Volume 18, Issue 10, pg. 687–689, December 1998

35. Bigal, M. Sheftell, F. Rapoport, A. Tepper, S. Lipton, R. Chronic Daily Headache: Identification of Factors Associated With Induction and Transformation. Headache: The Journal of Head and Face Pain Volume 42, Issue 7, pgs 575–581, July 2002.

36. United States Department of Agriculture (USDA). Agricultural Research Service. 2015. http://ars.usda.gov/News/docs.htm?docid=10874

37. Demirbilek H, Kandemir N, Gonc EN, Ozon A, Alikasifoglu A, Yordam N. Hashimoto's thyroiditis in children and adolescents: a retrospective study on clinical, epidemiological and laboratory properties

of the disease. Journal of Pediatric Endocrinology and   Metabolism. 2007 Nov;20(11):1199-205

38. Arrieta, MC, Bistritz, L, Meddings, JB. Alterations in intestinal permeability. Gut. 2006; 55(10): 1512-1520.

39. Koyuncu A, Aydintu S, Koçak S, Aydin C, Demirer S, Topçu O, Kuterdem E. Effect of thyroid hormones on stress ulcer formation. ANZ Journal of Surgery. 2002 Sep;72(9):672-5.

40. American Chiropractic Association. 2015. http://www.acatoday.org/level2_css.cfm?T1ID=13&T2ID=68

41. Paluszynska DA, Harris KA, Thach BT. Influence of sleep position experience on ability of prone-sleeping infants to escape from asphyxiating microenvironments by changing head position. Pediatrics. 2004 Dec;114(6):1634-9.

42. Majnemer, A. Barr, R. Association between sleep position and early motor Development. The Journal of Pediatrics. November 2006.Volume 149, Issue 5, Pages 623–629.e1

43. Hansraj, K. Assessment of Stresses in the Cervical Spine Caused by Posture and Position of the Head. Surgical Technology International. 2014.

44. Schilling, DL. Washington, K. Billingsley, F. Deitz, J. Classroom Seating for Children

with Attention Deficit Hyperactivity Disorder: Therapy Balls Versus Chairs. American Journal of Occupational Therapy, September/October 2003, Vol. 57, 534-541.

45. Liew, Z. Ritz, B. Rebordosa, C. Lee, PC. Acetaminophen Use During Pregnancy, Behavioral Problems, and Hyperkinetic Disorders. JAMA Pediatrics. April 2014, Vol 168, No. 4 .

46. Vaccine Injury. 2015. http://www.vaccineinjury.info/vaccinations-in-general/health-unvaccinated-children/survey-results-illnesses.html

47. Waly, M. Olteanu, H. Banerjee, R. Activation of methionine synthase by insulin-like growth factor-1 and dopamine: a target for neurodevelopmental toxins and thimerosal. Molecular Psychiatry (2004) 9, 358–370.

48. Exley, C. Vickers,T. Elevated brain aluminium and early onset Alzheimer's disease in an individual occupationally exposed to aluminium: a case report. 10 February 2014. Journal of Medical Case Reports 2014, 8:41

49. Bauer, A. Kriebel, D. Prenatal and Perinatal analgesic and Autism: and ecological link. 2013. Environmental Health. 12: 41.

50. Shaw,W. Evidence that Increased Acetaminophen use in Genetically Vulnerable Children Appears to be a Major Cause of the Epidemics of Autism, Attention Deficit with Hyperactivity, and Asthma. 2013. Journal of Restorative Medicine; 2: page 1-16

51. McCann, D. Berrett, A. Cooper, A, Crumpler, D. Food additives and hyperactive behaviour in 3-year-old and 8/9-year-old children in the community: a randomised, double-blinded, placebo-controlled trial. Nov. 2007. The Lancet. Volume 370, No. 9598, p1560–1567

52. Hill, I. Fasano, A. Schwartz, R. Counts, D. Glock, M. Horvath, K. The prevalence of celiac disease in at-risk groups of children in the United States. January 2000Volume 136, Issue 1, Pages 86–90.

53. Niederhofer, H. Association of Attention-Deficit/Hyperactivity Disorder and Celiac Disease: A Brief Report. 2011. The Primary Care Companion for CNS Disorders. 13(3).

54. Young,S. How to increase serotonin in the human brain without drugs. Nov. 2007. Journal of Psychiatry and Neuroscience. 32(6): 394-399.

55. Johnson, R. Gold, M. Johnson, D. Ishimoto,T. Attention-Deficit/Hyperactivity Disorder: Is it Time to Reappraise the Role

of Sugar Consumption? Sept. 2011. Postgraduate Medicine. 123(5): 39-49.

56. Stevens, L. Zentall, S. Abate, M. Kuczek, T. Burges, J. Omega-3 fatty acids in boys with behavior, learning, and health problems. Physiology & Behavior. April/May 1996. Volume 59, Issues 4–5, Pages 915–920.

57. Bilici M, Yildirim F, Kandil S, Bekaroğlu M, Yildirmiş S, Değer O, Ulgen M, Yildiran A, Aksu H. Double-blind, placebo-controlled study of zinc sulfate in the treatment of attention deficit hyperactivity disorder. Progress in Neuro-psychopharmacol and Biological Psychiatry. 2004 Jan;28(1):181-90.

58. Dodig-Curković K, Dovhanj J, Curković M, Dodig-Radić J, Degmecić D. The role of zinc in the treatment of hyperactivity disorder in children. Acta Medica Croatica. 2009 Oct;63(4):307-13.

59. Kamal, M. Is High Prevalence of Vitamin D Deficiency a Contributory Factor for Attention Deficit Hyperactivity Disorder in Children and Adolescents? June 9, 2014. ADHD Attention Deficit and Hyperactivity Disorders. 6(2): 73-8

60. Garland, C. Garland, F. Gorham, E. The Role of Vitamin D in cancer prevention. American Public Health Association. Feb. 2006. 96(2): 252-261.

61. Garland CF, Gorham ED, Mohr SB, Garland FC. Vitamin D for cancer prevention: global perspective. July 2009. Annals of Epidemiology. 19(7):468-83.

62. Alcantara J, Davis J. The chiropractic care of children with attention-deficit/hyperactivity disorder: a retrospective case series. Explore (NY). May-June 2010. 6(3):173-82.

63. International Chiropractic Pediatric Association. 2015. http://icpa4kids.org/Chiropractic-Research/ADD/ADHD/

64. Mysels, D. Sullivan, M. The relationship between opioid and sugar intake. Review of evidence and clinical applications. Journal of Opioid Management. 2010 ; 6(6): 445–452.

65. Colantuoni C1, Schwenker J, McCarthy J, Rada P, Ladenheim B, Cadet JL, Schwartz GJ, Moran TH, Hoebel BG. Excessive sugar intake alters binding to dopamine and mu-opioid receptors in the brain. Neuroreport. 2001 Nov 16;12(16):3549-52.

66. Deng, X. Song, Y. Manson, Signorello, Z. et al. Magnesium, vitamin D status and mortality: results from US National Health and Nutrition Examination Survey (NHANES) 2001 to 2006 and NHANES III. 2013. Biomed Central. 11:187.

67. Food and Drug Administration. 2015.
http://www.fda.gov/ohrms/dockets/ac/02
/briefing/3882b2_02_mcneil-
nsaid.htm#_Toc18761781

68. Sordillo, J, Scirica, C. Et al. Prenatal and
infant exposure to acetaminophen and
ibuprofen and the risk for wheeze and
asthma in children. The Journal of Allergy
and Clinical Immunology. February 2015.
Volume 135, Issue 2, Pages 441–448

69. Anrig, C. Plaugher, G. Pediatric
Chiropractic. 2013. Lippincott Williams &
Wilkins.

70. Center for Disease Control and Prevention.
April 2015. Centers for Disease Control
and Prevention Epidemiology and
Prevention of Vaccine-Preventable
Diseases, 13th Edition. www.cdc.gov

71. Yasko, A. Mullan, N. Gastrointestinal
Balance and Neurotransmitter Formation.
AUTISM SCIENCE DIGEST: THE JOURNAL OF
AUTISMONE. ISSUE 04

72. Schwalfenberg, G. The Alkaline Diet. Is
there Evidence that an Alkaline pH Diet
Benefits Health? Journal of Environmental
and Public Health. 2012.

73. Arnett, T. Regulation of bone cell function
by acid–base balance. Proceedings of
the Nutrition Society / Volume 62 / Issue 02
/ May 2003, pp 511-520

74. Klougart N, Nilsson N, Jacobsen J. Infantile Colic Treated by Chiropractors: A Prospective Study of 316 Cases. J Manipulative Physiol Ther 1989 (Aug); 12 (4): 281–288

75. Cowling, BJ, Et al. Increased risk of non-influenza respiratory virus infections associated with receipt of inactivated influenza vaccine. Clinical Infectious Diseases (2012)

76. doi: 10.1093/cid/cis307

77. Center for Disease Control and Prevention. 2015. Vaccine Effectiveness - How Well Does the Flu Vaccine Work? http://www.cdc.gov/flu/about/qa/vaccineeffect.htm

78. National Vaccine Information Center. 03.02.2011. No Pharma Liability? No Vaccine Mandates. http://www.nvic.org/NVIC-Vaccine-News/March-2011/No-Pharma-Liability--No-Vaccine-Mandates-.aspx

79. Supreme Court of the United States. Russell Bruesewitz et al v. Wyeth et al. No. 09-152. Argued October 12, 2010 – Decided February 22, 2011.

80. Center for Disease Control and Prevention. 2015. Past Immunization Schedules. http://www.cdc.gov/vaccines/schedules/past.html

81. PhRMA. 2015. Nearly 300 Vaccines in Development for Prevention and Treatment of Disease. http://www.phrma.org/media/releases/nearly-300-vaccines-development-prevention-treatment-disease

82. Steingraber, S. The Falling Age of Puberty in US Girls. 2007. Breast Cancer Fund. Pg. 52-58.

83. Alcantara, J. The successful chiropractic care of pediatric patients with chronic constipation: A case series and selective review of the literature. Clinical Chiropractic. Volume 11, Issue 3, September 2008, Pages 138–147

84. Ito, T., Jensen, R. Association of Long-term Proton Pump Inhibitor Therapy with Bone Fractures and effects on Absorption of Calcium, Vitamin B12, Iron, and Magnesium. Curr Gastroenterol Rep. 2010 Dec; 12(6): 448–457.

85. Towbin, A. Latent Spinal Cord and Brain Stem Injury in Newborn Infants. Develop Med Child Neurol, 1969; 11(1):54-68

86. Clum, D. The Magic Salt Sock: Natural Relief for Ear Infections. http://snoqualmievalley.macaronikid.com/article/636813/the-magic-salt-sock-natural-relief-for-ear-infections.

87. Louis, C. Scrutiny for Laxatives as a

Childhood Remedy. New York Times. 01.05.15 www.nytimes.com/2015/01/06/science/scrutiny-for-a-childhood-remedy.html?_r=0

88. Hollis, BW, et al. Maternal Versus Infant Vitamin D Supplementation During Lactation: A Randomized Controlled Trial. Pediatrics. 2015 Oct;136(4):625-34

Pictures by:

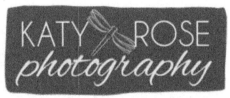

MATERNITY . BIRTH . NEWBORN . FAMILY

Coming Soon!

Be on the lookout for Dr. Brenda's next book on preparing for pregnancy and beyond.

The book will cover: preconception (preparing body for pregnancy), fertility, pregnancy, labor, and the 4th trimester, talking about everything from the importance of taking the right prenatal vitamins, thyroid, adrenal health during conception, diet, breastfeeding, Webster Chiropractic Technique, dangers of some over the counter medications, how to avoid lip tie and tongue tie, co-sleeping, and so much more.

If you are preparing for a little one, you will want to read this book!

Made in the USA
Middletown, DE
12 March 2019